The Day the Music Stopped

Re-enchantment of our lost spirit

Beverlee Zell-Tamis, Ph.D.

CARLISLE PRESS

Published by Carlisle Press in association with Tenacity Press. Inquiries should be addressed to Carlisle Press. Phone: 520-282-6862. Email: Beverleesee4ever@aol.com.

Grateful acknowledgment is given for permission to reprint excerpts from:

The Glass Bead Game (Magister Ludi) by Hermann Hesse. © 1943 by Fretz and Wasmuth Verlag AG, Zurich. English translation © 1969 by Holt, Rinehart & Winston; © 1990 Henry Holt and Company. Reprinted by permission of Henry Holt and Company. LLC.

"I Have Longed to Move Away," by Dylan Thomas, from *The Poems of Dylan Thomas.* © 1939 by New Directions Publishing Corp. Reprinted by permission of New Directions Publishing Corp.

Library of Congress Cataloging-in Publication Data

Zell-Tamis, Beverlee
The day the music stopped: re-enchantment of our lost spirit /
Beverlee Zell-Tamis. — 1st ed.
p. cm.
Includes bibliographical references.
ISBN 1-892193-08-6 (pbk.)
1. Self — Edited tapes. 2. Pain — Psychological aspects — Edited tapes.
3. Suffering — Edited tapes. 4. Spiritual life — Edited tapes. 5. Self-actualization— (Psychology) — Edited tapes.
I. Title.
BF697.Z45 2000
158—dc21 00-037703

Cover design: Marc Tamis
Cover photo: Ron Johnson with Susan J. Sparrow
Cover color photo: Peter W. Stearns from *Mendocino County Wildflowers*

Printed and bound in the United States of America

9 7 5 3 1 2 4 6 8 10

Dedicated with Love to
Robert, Lisa, and Brant

ACKNOWLEDGMENTS

I always believed it would be difficult to include everyone who had influenced my life and especially this book. Like my life this book is a journey and the destination is not known. Many have been present giving time, effort, support, loving critique, and by their nature diminished the anxiety and loneliness of writing.

My deeply abiding thank you to my husband for hours of typing edited script into computer form and always encouraging the worth of my written words; to my editor Hal Zina Bennett whose thoughtful questions and knowledge enabled the best of me to step up to a daunting task of writing a book about the self; to the voices who risked sharing their core person and beautifully enhanced the text; to Susan J Sparrow for her creativity and labor in bringing this book to fruition; to Phyllis Arthur who began the project with me spending hours finding books in the library and typing my original manuscript; to Lyn Stimer and Norma Gurovitch who encouraged and supported my work; to Eugene Berman, a life-long friend, who became a needed reader and critic; to Amanda Bauman who entered all handwritten material into a computer; to Barbara Stalling who transcribed hours and hours of dialogue with the ten voices; to Karen Heard for her artistic input on the cover concept; to friends and fellow writers whose encouragement and knowledge kept me going when words failed; and finally to my mother and father who shared their wonder, humor, and curiosity of life which lives on as my spiritual guide.

CONTENTS

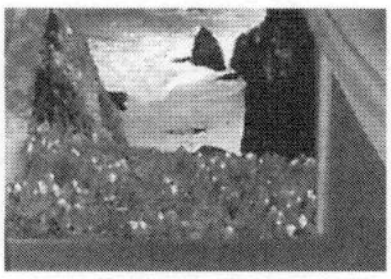

Introduction

Frozen silence...Darkness prevails on darkness.
One shaft of light breaks through the jagged clouds
Coming from Nothingness to penetrate the depths,
Compound the night with day, build length and breadth,
Prefigure peak and ridge, declivities, redoubts,
A loose blue atmosphere, earth's deep dense fullness.

That brilliant shaft dissevers teeming generation
Into both deed and war, and in a frenzy of creation
Ignites a gleaming terrified new world.
All changes where the seeds of light descend,
Order arises, magnificence is heard
In praise of life, of victory to light's great end.

The mighty urge glides on, to move
Its power into all creatures' being,
Recalling far divinity, the spirit of God's doing:
Now joy and pain, words, art, and song,
World towering on world in arching victory throng
With impulse, mind, contention, pleasure, love.

HERMANN HESSE[1]

When I thought about the struggle of my life and about the struggles of other people I had known, I knew that I would need to write this book. Like lines in the palm of my hand, my relationships had touched, crossed, and withstood the pressure of time. Some connections were brief, others became friendships that lasted for years. Those who cared for me, and I them, my dearest relations, enriched my soul beyond measure.

When I began this book, my mind, heart, and hand reached out to locate by phone these old friends. I asked to meet and tape-record in-depth conversations about our lives. As we visited, their stories told to me were both mysterious and exciting. The ten tapings were remarkable because they echoed similar themes. I felt in some way that I had not lost touch, that communication had been continuous even when it hadn't seemed to be. The energies of our lives were invested in similar and different paths.

In this book I refer to these edited tapes as *voices* since they speak truly in their own words. They reflected many thoughts, many moods, many feelings: anxiety and fear, joy and sadness, anger, warmth, and love. They reflected on who they had been, who they had become, and the dreary and wonderful scenarios of their lives. Even as I wrote and recorded their stories I knew that what they told me was valuable information.

I was drawn to several common themes. At the center of our core personality there appeared to be holes, that is, damaged parts of ourselves, or perhaps a void, a missing part, something about us that became a source of enormous displeasure. I knew each of us believed we had fallen short of our ideal self during certain periods of our lives. At times our voids were apparent, at other times less visible, but always lurking somewhere within us. Sometimes the voids were understood by me and the ten *voices* as failings or deficits which had damaged our productive choices. I saw the holes or voids as a Swiss cheese phenomena of the psyche.

In my life I had tried over many years to permanently fill my voids. Frustration and anxiety signaled a spectacular lack of success, because the voids never permanently disappeared. I did not know then that these deficits are also blessings. Certainly, there were periods of happiness, joy, adventure, achievement, and sharing. But what was this nagging lack of confidence, or at times, feelings of negativity and failed expectations? Why did I periodically fall into a hole larger than the self I respected? There were times, I will share later, when my life was moving along and suddenly the bottom dropped out. Why when all things seemed comfortable and settled did the world turn suddenly cold? Why did the music stop, the energy die?

I had taken out the pieces of the puzzle hundreds of times and I was able to fit together some of the parts. I believed that when I assembled the puzzle — the colorful pieces of my life — I would have a knowledge of the origin of my deficits and therefore the voids would never resurface. I believed the music would play forever. I expected that my life in the middle years would achieve harmony and peacefulness. That was not to be. My midlife contained some of the most turbulent times, even though many structures were in place: marriage, career, family, artistic creation.

Over the years of being a psychotherapist, many people have shared important aspects of their lives with me. Whether they spoke of their conscious ego or their larger spiritual self, within a short period of time the sense of these voids or deficits became serious considerations for therapy. My life and theirs had a similar echo. Had the holes enlarged because of critical events in life? Did the music stop with no apparent cause like the sound of a radio when the station fades out?

I wanted to understand a mystery. What is the relationship, if any, between our original voids, the deficits we experience from birth, and subsequent events? Are these deficits alone responsible for our music diminishing or stopping? As I taped my friends' voices, all spoke about early wounds, some as far back as infancy. I knew even more clearly that none of us had escaped damaging experiences. My own turmoil reflected strong feelings about voids within myself. One large deficit had been ongoing anxiety and fear beginning as early as I could remember. It was a strange birthright and a birth death as well.

I stumbled upon a concept referred to as "compensatory structure." Heinz Kohut, an elderly German psychoanalyst, now deceased, wrote about the two parts of compensatory structure: aims, goals, and ambitions, and ideals. Our aims, goals, and ambitions are of major importance and are activated during our adult years in the form of work, love, play, and creativity. Ideals, the second part of compensatory structure, are the values, standards of behavior, and principles of living we accept and strive to achieve. Certainly, it made sense that my original self-deficit, the Swiss cheese of my psyche, should greatly affect the choices and success of my goals and ideals.

The patterns and themes of work, love, and play expressed by the friends I interviewed, as well as the lives of those I guided in therapy, started me on a quest to find any common elements woven through our life tapestries. I wanted to shed some light on the complex and painful phenomenon of feeling defective, of losing spirit, and more importantly, *how we restored what we had lost, how we had built vital compensatory structures.* Why do apparently self-confident, accomplished human beings fall into a dark hole, which for a time snatches away important meaning in their lives? Just at the moment when everything appears to be going so well, a demon arrives creating doubt, pain, confusion. When life events are destructive and chaotic the demon punishes with even more terror. The music stops. You have heard the expression "get a life." But what happens when more than once, you have a life and you wake up and all you feel is a quiet, dead feeling or agitated anxiety? You may ask yourself if you are depressed. Few, if any, of the symptoms of depression are present. If this loss of spirit is not depression as we clinically understand it, then we need to solve our mystery. Why did our music stop?

I knew I would share, in book form, some beliefs, some theoretical ideas, and some thoughts, which had repeated over and over in my mind. We are *all* products to some degree of a dysfunctional or disinterested family — one without healthy energy for a particular child. In our early lives we were *born with* and *developed* deficits and voids. Our self-deficit created wounds and often we felt guilt or shame during different phases of our life. When we saw parts of ourselves as defective, our balance sheet would register a zero and, as a result, we held in our hands an empty promise to trust ourself. Without trust, our confidence and self esteem plummeted. Finally, our authentic essence, the truest energy of our spirit may be lost. Work, play, and love relationships — the most important forms of goals and ideals - alive at one moment, disappear, and even appear dead to us. On that day, our music stops, the sound inaudible.

I have come to believe, to see that for most of us a path to restoring our authentic self is possible. A way to be, to think, to understand, and to act exists to restore our dislocated and lost self. Transformative work, play, love, creativity, humor, relationships, and discovery of our true self becomes the path of our restoration, our re-enchantment.

We alone can provide an inner space which is non-judgmental and unconditionally loving. We are not here only to be molded by family and society, we are here to impact those who come after us just by being our best self. We can transmute and reclaim the design of our deepest spirit in such a form that it brings creativity and bliss to ourselves and all those around us. We can become richer beings, both aware and comfortable with powerful transitions, and we have choice and freedom to accomplish those things that provide us with a joyful, exuberant existence. *Re-enchanted, transcendent beings are those who discover their richer material, prima materia, and they know the heart of their personal mystery.*

"People should tell their own stories and own their own memory."[2] In an effort to honor my peers, friends, and colleagues I have, with their permission, given them a voice in this book. They have shared painful and difficult experiences. To open the doors to their memories is a courageous act and I am deeply grateful to them for contributing their essence and wisdom. My friends' *voices* represent a vitality of identity only they could provide. Their perceptions and light have vastly enriched the themes of this book and have forever changed and transformed my life as well. Their tapes, hours of sometimes emotional dialogue with me, have been shortened but their truth is present and clear.

A friend, in speaking about the work I am doing, referred to it as a psychology book. Without thinking, I said, "this writing is about myself." It is a piece of me but it is also a piece of all those to whom I've been connected, as Native Americans say, "to all my relations." What I select, what I exclude, what I research, what I decide to punctuate, what takes form and what is necessary can only be in its deepest essence my journal, my subjective awareness of all I know and all I do not know.

The process of writing is not as I imagined: words beckon to me, books beckon to me. I am pulled and pushed by forces I don't always understand. Friends no longer participating in my life beckon to me. I've allowed my inner spirit to follow intuitive instructions and I've opened myself to hearing and seeing all that I can. I have opened the door to my unconscious. I have opened my heart.

My deepest desire was to contribute "a truth" to my fellow beings. All of us share a heritage; we incorporate experiences that damage our souls. We are fragmented by these. We struggle courageously to build, to compensate, to heal, to find worth and meaning and to restore our lost spirit. We do this in the context of another - you and me committed to a dialogue, or at least imaginary conversations.

From birth to death, there are no immune systems that protect us from forming voids and walking or leaping into them. But we who have experienced serious wounds are able to restore our lost spirits. The most seriously damaged beings amongst us can create new and different themes of work, love, and play and can find our richer, deeper essence after falling into deep, cavernous holes.

We don't die with all the wounds healed but at the end we need to know we have worked always toward the light, toward some restoring of our self. David Geffen, the powerful head of a large music conglomerate speaks: "We all die unhealed, we all acquire damage as infants and children and we work on removing those scars all of our lives. You won't heal everything, but what's important is the work. I'm a great believer in anything that makes you one percent better. So I try everything."[3]

During critical periods of my life my voids widen, deepen, drag me down kicking and screaming. I am encapsulated by fearful internal and external experiences. In fact, I knew fear from the very beginning of my life. My mother and father had multiple fears and anxieties. Taking them on was easy.

I do not expect to have my energy restored, to be safe at one moment in time and have this safety last forever. I am challenged at all times. I experience the good work of my life and the meaning I attribute to it as a progression of paths. I complete some paths but new paths constantly challenge me.

I AM FOREVER WALKING.

What appears to be a terrible thought, that I cannot create a stable, permanently healed self is in reality a blessing. I cannot live without my deficits, my demons, my fears; they awaken passionate needs to live fully, to be totally present as a divine, authentic essence. I am not the walking dead.

Now and again we catch a glimpse of something that transcends the daily struggle, something that transforms our soul's destiny. We are lifted to awareness, to recognition that is beyond the mindset of satisfying ego demands. We catch a glimpse of our own transcendence, our richer truth. We seek restoration. We reclaim our soul's energy. *We hear the music.*

It is a challenge and responsibility of our life to provide joy, creativity, goals, and vitality. It is a challenge to provide an authentic self, to provide the music of our soul. It is a challenge to exist in this world, accepting change, accepting risk, accepting vulnerability, accepting ourselves just as we are. I hope that this journey the *voices* and I share with you will provide hope and courage during your quest for a richer, more joyful life.

Notes to the Introduction

1. Hermann Hesse, *The Glass Bead Game, Magister Ludi* (New York: Holt, Rinehart & Winston, Inc., 1969), p. 403.
2. Salvador Minuchin and Charles H. Fishman, *Family Therapy Techniques* (Cambridge, MA: Harvard University Press, 1983).
3. David Geffen, *New York Times Sunday Magazine of the Week Section.* 5/2/93.

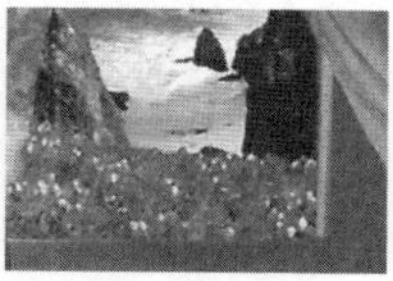

CHAPTER 1

The Day the Music Stopped

If I am not for myself — who will be?
If I am only for myself — what am I?
If not now — when?

HILLEL (*SONG OF OUR FATHERS*)[1]

DO YOU RECALL THE DAY the music stopped? The terror, days of silence, not knowing how many mornings you would awaken to nothingness. Before this your life may have moved swiftly along in a goal-directed fashion. Perhaps choices were made that were ambitious as you met short-term and long-term goals. Initiative and motivation to perform any and all tasks felt good as you ran to your accepted destiny. You climbed the mountain of achievements, both career and personal relationships, and enough gains and rewards occurred to match your best efforts. All the time you heard some music playing and felt joy as each of your aims succeeded.

Now there is a deadly silence or a faint sound off in the distance. You are, perhaps, any age — twenty or thirty, forty or fifty, or sixty. Friends may see some changes; you are immobilized, unhappy, frightened, anxious. Your confusion is all the more painful because your life represents goals you have chosen. Depression doesn't seem to be what you are experiencing. Something else has occurred — the music stopped!

In my life I have always connected to specific goals, and yet my music periodically stops. When I entered Smith College, I knew my major would be psychology. My curiosity about people's lives existed from childhood, I was forever asking questions and was nicknamed the "lawyer." Now an opportunity in college existed to really understand human nature. My troubled self was at the heart of a need to discover anything and everything about humans.

After college, this craving in psychology was put on hold as I became wife, mother, teacher, artist, real estate sales person, etc., etc. Marriage, divorce, new marriage, the years running away. There were frequent intrusive thoughts about graduate school and a return to education. But some rewards existed as each different path reflected my inner voice, funding my soul with space for creative outlets — painting, sculpting in stone, writing letters. I let the years run their course without demanding something more. During these years I experienced times of despair — sometimes it was associated with unhappy events such as my divorce and being a single mother — but there were times when relatively little was damaging. My life was active and then . . . the music would stop, my energy dying.

In my forties there was a crisis. I formed a partnership with a friend and we became art consultants to large corporations. It was challenging to relate to corporate minds and artists' visions, farthest ends of a large continuum. It certainly felt joyful, the communication stimulating on many levels. Nothing seemed amiss. Three years passed. One morning I awoke and I knew the music had stopped. There was a profound, gloomy silence. I had an awareness of waves of anxiety. It was confusing, but my intuition told me nothing was going to stay the same. My personal and professional life would be tossed in the air like a ball.

It was a long time before my inner spirit sorted this out. Some things were dying. My true identity had not been acknowledged. My strong intuitive powers weren't ready to know or deal with the death. Art consulting finally brought me to an edge of boredom. My marriage was failing, and I felt despair. The cavern of old voids opened, yawned wider into a lack of trust in myself, and filled me with fear and anxiety. I was engulfed by a major dislocation of my spirit. I was lying in my bed like someone who had a near drowning. Here I was in the most productive years of my life unable to hear my music. Later, perhaps weeks later, an intuitive glimmer would bring me to some truth, a strong internal need to return to graduate school, an awakening to visions of being a therapist, using my dormant resources and skills. By then it was a clear necessity and I would have to get out of bed to begin to accomplish this. That was years ago, and now I am turning inward once again, discovering a new road for restoring my spirit's energy. The stories of the voices and I reside in the pages that follow; our paths as anxious, dislocated spirits becoming transcendent beings is everyone's journey. Eleven of us will share with you intimate life experiences.

Each of you may have produced, or been unable to produce, your own unique and creative life. Each of you may have been silenced for a time during your best years or perhaps you did not hear your music at all. How and why did this chosen life at various points in time become pained, faulty, or useless? What perceptions did you have of what was possible? What was the meaning of your life, love, family, work, creativity, relationship? Was the most important game worth playing primarily your career and job? Were your daily choices things you loved to do?

What is the game now? In fact, do you have a game worth playing? Was the meaning of your life something more than all the daily experiences of living?

Shana's story shares the frustration of an early belief in what was a worthy game, namely, marriage and family. She expected to share her music with her spouse. In her words, she thought that the "Disney kid belief in a happy life with a husband" would be enough for her spirit. Over time her beliefs, growth, and choices overwhelmed this vision. She required more than that relationship to have her music play. As we follow her story, Shana slowly develops several themes, several games worth playing. At the age of twenty-two she began a quest for more information about her interior, multi-dimensional being; she was asking, who or what could acknowledge her essence, restore her balance?

Shana's mother-in-law gave her an unintended picture of what the Disney life would be. Although Shana liked her mother-in-law and maintained a connection until the older woman died, she was aware that she could not live the same kind of life. The Sunday dinner was a metaphor for the woman's roles as only a nurturer, cook, housekeeper, and family-oriented being. The routine of every Sunday dinner, the sameness, created terror in Shana.

> **SHANA: I was about twenty-two when it came to a crisis. I looked around and two things happened. One Sunday, we walked into [my husband's] parents' house . . . we would go over and share dinner. They would watch football games. From the first time I met my former mother-in-law, we were so deeply connected . . . but I walked in there one Sunday and it hit me so profoundly that if my husband and I continued the way we were, this is what I could look forward to when I was sixty years old. This was**

exactly the circumstance, the setting, the kind of relationship, the family . . . I almost broke out in hives! There is no way to explain the kind of impact that this had. It was a total message from within, which was: "Wake up! Pay attention! This will have to change." I was still coming from the orientation that here I am, a good wife. I have a good husband, we have a good home, we accomplish things together. "Shana, what's wrong with you?" That you could look at this picture and say, "No." Something's vibrating saying, "This will have to change. This will have to be done differently." It really terrified me.

I remember so clearly standing in the kitchen saying this to my husband and I was absolutely sobbing, "I'm so unhappy. I am so miserable. I'm twenty-two years old, I have a wonderful husband, who is definitely devoted. I have a beautiful, healthy son. I have a lovely, comfortable home. It's the proverbial two cars in the garage and the husband who comes home from work every day. Everything is there and I am miserable." I even said to him, "I have everything that I thought I wouldn't get until I was fifty years old and I am miserable." Which of course, he also couldn't understand.

I grew up as a Disney Kid! What I mean is that there is a fairy tale overlay. When I finally decided to get married . . . I was going to be able to finally tell him EVERYTHING I had cataloged, stored, put in closets, in safety. Of course he would totally understand all this and at last I would be able to just say, "What about this perspective?" Or, you know, "I've always thought this about that." That's not what happened. He recoiled! He recoiled in such a way that his response was, "My God, Shana, what's wrong with you?" I realized that deep inside, what that meant was this particular being would never be capable of understanding even a fraction of me.

I just shut down. I just started pulling myself, my beingness, back in. What I ended up feeling like was a person within a person . . . what the roles are . . . wife and daughter, mother and business person, and all the rest of that. I will give those roles my absolute commitment because I certainly care about this man. The roles led to cycles of feeling dead, numb, but also anger, fear, and sadness . . . anger, fear, and grief, those I've certainly come to understand, those are the three issues.

I performed. Absolutely I did. My mother had been tremendously abused as a child, and so had my father. Yet, they made very clear what I considered to be strong, committed, courageous choices to stop that process. And they did! The message they sent me was that all things are truly possible. You may have to work very hard. There may be other things you have to give up for that to happen.

I started creating other interests or attempting to bring in other stimulation into our relationship. How do you fix it? What can I do? Surely, if I'm the one that is seeing the insight, then that must mean it's my job to fix it. So I sought out therapists. "What's wrong with me?" It's got to be something I'm not doing.

The beauty for me was following the inner voice. I stepped up and asked for help when I got to whatever my point of pain was. When I went in for the session, I really thought that someone, who knew better than I, would tell me how to fix it. We'll go through the little dance, move our arms, legs, hands, feet or whatever. I'll start wearing turtlenecks instead of crewnecks, and they lived happily ever after.

One of the things the therapist told me was that he wasn't going to fix me. My first reaction to that was, "See? Not only is there something wrong with you, it can't even be fixed."

One of the things I did was I used my creativity, whether it was making clothing or things like art pieces that went on the wall. I did go back and forth to work. I did have bridges where I would go in and out. It gave me an outlet that was very rich and very important.

But over time not enough! The message from Shana's parents was simple: you can make anything work. But in a major way, this life Shana chose did not fit her spiritual or personal needs. Eventually she shut down. Her multi-leveled personality couldn't continue an unshared existence with a fixed, rigid husband who did not have a clue about the spiritual reality of this person he lived with every day. There was a poor fit. No way for them to change: no way to "fix" it: no way to maintain harmony or feel joy.

Many of you question, just as Shana did, what being happy is all about or how to fulfill your needs, both personal and spiritual. Csikszentmihalyi, in his book *Flow,* directly addresses questions about happiness and the conditions necessary for enjoying optimal experiences in our lives. Love, work, play, and creativity are necessary, but our joyful essence, as Csikszentmihalyi would say, is something else. It is a state of being, to fully experience the moment, allowing passion now as you pursue your life dreams.

Focus is a key element for me. I ski, I ski hard and fast, or I ski with reverence for the snow gently conforming my motions to each bend and turn. My concentration is always present as I transverse down the slope, but my choice of hard or gentle is a way of being, an environment I have created on my way down the mountain.

Bliss demands my deepest concentration as it requires me to immerse myself in goals or events with such verve that optimal experience is created. This dedication to life is called *Flow.* For me it is like completing a marble sculpture and feeling a sense of rapture when I do my work. All that I need is contained within the experience; I don't require external rewards under these circumstances. In the years that I sculpted, each time I placed the air hammer point or chisel against the stone and ground it into the newly created form, a sense of wonder and excitement filled me. I knew in a mysterious way what was coming. The chisel would seemingly move by itself to different sections. At some point it was time to use files, water, and sandpaper to create a completely smooth finish. Throughout the process a final form remained in my mind's eye. My hands would go over the stone hundreds of times, checking for rough spots. When the sculpture was finished, I knew intuitively to release the water and carefully wipe dry each section. As I turned the piece around several times to see all that existed, a sense of awe overwhelmed me. I had created this!

What is the common ground which describes a flow experience? "It provided a sense of discovery, a creative feeling of transporting the person into a new reality. It pushed the person to higher levels of performance, and led to previously undreamed of states of consciousness."[2] Yes, that definition describes the mystery and nourishment available when I pierced a marble stone and discovered a form of beauty hidden deep, deep within.

At the same time that I was sculpting I formed my art consulting business with a fellow artist. I believed that the easy flow and happiness of my life could continue. This art business became successful early on because no one else at that time provided corporate art collections and creative installations. In three years we explored all the interesting connections necessary to build art collections for corporate and professional companies. But my intense need to be invested with people on a more complex, challenging, intimate level ate away my feeling of joy. Art consulting developed a sameness to all the daily elements and soon I had no time for sculpting. I lost my source of creativity. My spiritual energy was dying. Being happy was impossible.

If passion, discovery, creativity is missing in your life, is there a way to focus on events and people which create optimal experiences? Strangely enough the most despairing, crisis-ridden time of life does, by its nature, push and pull you, bringing your attention to goals and life visions that become clear and unchallenged the more you focus on them. You may be muddling along with vague aims, discontent activity, unvitalized projects and obsolete jobs, when suddenly, a severe crisis punctuates the path you must travel. The crisis forces you to your last bastion, yourself and your essential needs. Perhaps at the end of hope, you are forced to channel energy directly to your intuitive power. There is nowhere else to go, nothing more to lose. Different dreams and ideals surface. You gain an awareness that your life must change and you are capable of changing it. You may feel a serious longing for new experiences and a desire for every small, creative step that will provide optimal experiences, your music. Creating change, accepting transitions, is almost impossible *if you have not been in pain or experienced a crisis.* It is surely an irony of life that when you are in pain, you create your music. In this sense, pain and the demons are gifts. Many of us would turn down this gift of pain if we could. At the time you are fired from your work, you say "don't let this happen. I feel devastated." But being fired often opens new doors to creating work closer to your essense.

Another problem may exist. The identities you maintain — mother, father, daughter, son, working peer, social friend, family advisor on and on — grow more demanding. These "chairs" that you sit in occupy more than 100 percent of you, corrupting your ability to sit joyfully in each place. Everything runs into everything else. If you cannot balance the time in each identity that you assume, or in each chair that you choose, the music dies. A profound dislocation of the spirit tells you something isn't working, something is painfully out of balance.

In an unpublished paper Roy Doughty wrote:

> *We cannot go anywhere outside of ourselves to achieve balance. No time management course, no schedule juggling, no priority settings, no method at all can lead us out of ourselves.*
>
> *Things are out of balance because we are out of balance. We have to start in the midst of the mess and pay attention, not to what we should have done or must do, not to where we've been or would like to be, but to who we are right here, right now.*
>
> *My two-year-old daughter knew (without words) that the secret of inner continuity is outward attentiveness to the moment. It is a state of flow that we all have experienced, but have trained ourselves to repress. Balance requires waking up to the minute task that is right in front of us.*
>
> *If the first step in achieving balance is realizing the inviolability of the self, the second is realizing the same state in others. When we feel ourselves being torn by either/or choices, we have to ask for others to support us in*

being in the moment, and we have to learn to give that support to them.[3]

Dougherty says his young daughter knows instinctively to pay attention to whatever is at hand. Small children do this easily. As adults we play so many roles, our days are fragmented. That is why we must give our best self to the choice immediately before us, to live in this moment, to enjoy the full essence of how it feels, smells, tastes, looks, moves, etc. Each identity has its own time, and space. When my grandson, age five, visited recently at Thanksgiving, we built a large wooden plane, took time to paint it in the most joyful primary fluorescent colors — all of this during the busy preparation of a Thanksgiving feast. Grandy (me) will always see his colors next to each other, a parade of neon red, green, blue, yellow. Somehow it all flowed together, the total experience in a perfect sequence of visual joy.

Will searching and finding one or two areas of bliss be enough to provide all of our music? Perhaps, but not for most of us. One morning we may find our needs changing and awaken to a dying spirit.

A vital *series of ambitions and challenges* over the years and in many contexts of my life — work, play, love, relationship — created the spark that caused me to feel wonderfully alive. All of the elements of joyfulness are woven, unwoven, rewoven many times over like a tapestry that is never finished. The importance is my participation in a series of ambitions that allowed change. My work choices included a sequence of careers, teaching, sales, art consulting, working artist, psychotherapist, writer. I was emotionally invested during each new career focus. However, my work as a psychotherapist has endured the longest because it challenged my mind and heart. It allowed me a mutual journey with those spirits whose systems were failing. It provides mysteries to be solved, as well as opportunities to be a guide to others. Together we found our creativity and inner true voice. For me being a therapist contained all the conditions of optimal experience, yet my life required many other elements as well. Not the least were friendship and family.

What remains constant, never lost, is the integrity and vitality of our lives as we add new themes. Where once we chose jobs and careers to last a lifetime, we can no longer accept roles that are unchallenging, boring, or which evoke deep distress to our bodies and spirits. We can learn to express our authentic essence. No more pain in the neck, wrench in the gut. For many of us, vitality is created when we expand our experiences. We see with an inner eye what is next to do. With some fear we take a leap of faith.

Are we responsible for protecting each choice that is compatible with our unique essence? Are we responsible for our own music? Yes, but! There appears to be no magic path given to us at birth that creates a strong inner voice and preserves our unique road. When we hear the *voices*, or tune in to our personal stories, we know that each of us is responsible for a do-it-yourself program. Ambitions and dreams differ wildly. Few of us choose the same instruments to create aliveness and joy. We struggle always for a foothold on a steep, slippery path.

Kay's story instructs us with a lovely metaphor, where the steep path and responsibility are at issue. There is no question that she has been assaulted by life's events; she cannot avoid her own Swiss cheese holes. How she responded to those experiences, what she chose, is the difference between a joyful acceptable game of life or an unhappy dead-end journey. I was especially touched by this story because my family could not provide an initial path or instruction to help me know the way. I had to seek different mentors since my young parents were themselves engaged in simply learning how to survive. Survive, they did. Survive, I did.

> KAY: My father taught me everything that I know. I was a very independent person. Although I didn't work, I had been arranging my own things for years.
>
> My father made my life very easy for me. When I was about sixteen, he said, "Now, Kay, before a person is born, you go before the dear Lord, and He gives you a little box. In this little box is everything that ever happens to a person — sadness, happiness, illness, riches, everything." He said we all have the same things in our box, only we have them in totally different proportions. "They're all just sitting there waiting to be something. They are like raw material. Your job in life is to take everything that's in the box and make it all work to a satisfactory conclusion." Then he said that you go back to the dear Lord and he will say to you, "Okay, what did you do with your box?" You set it down and say to Him, "I couldn't do anything with this box, it's such a terrible box. If I'd had so-and-so's box, she got this and that." He will say, "I'm not interested in so-and-so's box, all I'm interested in is what you did with your box." So you see, my whole life I had a one-track mind. I had a mind-set that I had my box and whatever happens, I'm responsible for making everything in this box work. And there is no woman's excuse. You are not allowed to say, "Well, I was not allowed to do that."
>
> My father said, "Now you're going to hate me at times. I'm going to make you responsible for everything that ever happens to you. There is a way to solve all problems and it's up to you to find it. If one way doesn't work, you find another."

So I came to my relationship with the idea that no matter what it was, I was going to make it work. I had to make a life for myself in which I could go to bed every night without being upset about anything. You earn it? Your whole life you don't know what you're going to come up against. As long as I tended to my box, it didn't matter.

The metaphor of "the box" created a specific perspective — Kay could direct choices knowing that all the parts would need to fit. She fully accepted responsibility to deal with much of life's chaos and tragedy. Kay's life included being born with a defect of the spine which caused pain and limitation. Her husband required special care after returning from the war with an obsessive disorder. Raising seven fiercely independent children presented many challenges as well. Her daughter Emily's story confirms the difficult environment in this family system of seven siblings. Later we learn more about Kay's box from her granddaughter, Cassi, who tells her own story in another chapter.

Kay's daughter and granddaughter are the recipients of a legacy. Their ancestors were a storehouse of vitality and creativity. Four generations of extraordinary women. Each has a unique box. Each found a way to take everything in their box and make it work, but not without serious challenges.

Although Kay's metaphor created a structure for responsibility and choice that fit beautifully with her life, others perceive responsibility in quite a different way. Responsibilities may weigh heavily on your spirit and overwhelm you. Some of that burden is a recognition that you are not able to follow spontaneously or joyfully several creative paths. More importantly if you do follow one, then there is a nagging voice saying you must give up something. The choices and trade-offs are clear in the following story, which I would like to share.

One evening after a lovely dinner, my husband and I sat around a fire with some old friends. One of the men was an extremely dedicated professional, known for spending long hours at the office. Suddenly, I heard him speak about his love of music, that he had sung operata and played the violin as a young man. He expressed sadness concerning his lack of time or energy to conduct these pursuits. I was astonished to hear this since he had never spoken about this part of his life.

As we talked about giving up the things we loved to do, I heard the lonely whistle of a missed train. He quickly acknowledged the importance of his career, the pleasure it had given him, and the self-esteem it engendered, but with one disclaimer: there were times in the last decade when the work had become tedious, sometimes boring, even exhausting. His work during this last year did not create enough joy to sustain him.

As we said goodnight, my thoughts were drawn to his dilemma, to his burdens. The game worth playing for thirty-five years had been his professional career. He had accomplished this with humor, with vitality, and with some joy in his daily life. The trade-off was relinquishing some things he loved to do, some things that had provided bliss. I could not question his choices, yet felt sadness with him for what he had left behind. My friend left some creative part of his soul without its time for expression. In a literal sense his music is gone. He reflected more about this loss as his career became more tiring and demanding, yet there appeared to be no deep regrets, only some loss of energy and his vague wish to reclaim his more creative spirit.

We all leave something we love behind us because we cannot do it all. Some trade-off must be accepted. I felt and heard the lonely whistle when I gave up sculpting alabaster and marble stone. Pain accompanied this necessary loss as I moved on to new energy invested in my next career.

If you reflect and ruminate about your current choices, you may encounter an unwelcome reflection. Your spirit may bear signs of atrophy or drying up, sounds similar to the crackles of very old parchment paper blown along a sidewalk. The vital authentic self, the creative identity themes of your divine essence may be withering. It is not that you abandoned your destiny. A careful attention directed you to goals and ambitions which included healthy choices of work, love, and play. Without full awareness you may have chosen these to fill some of the early deficits of self, those Swiss cheese holes we spoke about. Why did they weaken or disappear entirely?

My life represents one piece of the puzzle. Many of my decisions led to paths which contributed to my building a worthy self, and they were effective for a time. They enhanced my self-esteem and confidence. I felt I could play my unique music indefinitely. Now, in the distance, is the lonely sound of a train's whistle. My destiny has once again become mysteriously fragile. I sense a loss. I know from within that solutions along the way did not prevent me from experiencing this current withering of my soul. I no longer feel safe because those choices that worked for me during the past years no longer fit who I am. Time changes everyone. No environment stays the same. Everything in this world is changing rapidly and there is a fearful dislocation of my spirit. My black hole has opened up. I want to feel alive, vital, competent. There is a sense of mystery about my current collapse. I want to solve the mystery so that my life is once again passionate and meaningful. What I do know is that what worked before is no longer viable.

The acceptance of deep rooted self-alterations and transitions is at the heart of re-enchantment. We are at a place in our life and the bottom drops out, or a calm occurs. We become aware that nothing is moving. We may be stopped dead in our tracks or condemned to walking exhausting paths one upon another. The potential for movement exists, the series of choices awaits our attention and energy, yet everything remains only a potential.

Not only are transformations of the self healthy, they are essential to the survival of our authentic self. Birth to death is a long journey for many. In modern life living to ninety is not unusual. We must hear the inner voice of our soul now, for even its smallest change in sound gives us new directions.

What I remember most in the movie, *When Harry Met Sally,* were the tapes of interviews with elderly couples. They expressed tenderness, harmony, wisdom, empathic understanding, and humor as they briefly told their story of bonded, committed relationships. What the story and camera caught was the essence of integrity, independence, and natural wisdom of these wonderful elders. One senses that they created a series of games worth playing. Instinctively, I want to play the game, to share in the fun. I want them to tell me the secret. I want to know I can grow old with humor, joy, and dignity. I want to hear my music. I think we all do.

Notes to Chapter 1

1. Mishnah 14. "If I am not for myself, who is for me? And being only for my own self, what am I? And if not now, when?" Hillel, 10 B.C. Translated and annotated by Hyman E. Goldin. *Ethics of the Fathers* (Hebrew Publishing Company, New York, 1962)
2. Mihaly Csikszentmihalyi, *Flow, The Psychology of Optimal Experience* (New York: Harper & Row, 1990), p. 67.
3. Roy Doughty, unpublished paper, *Balance,* p. 1, p. 2, pp. 3–4.

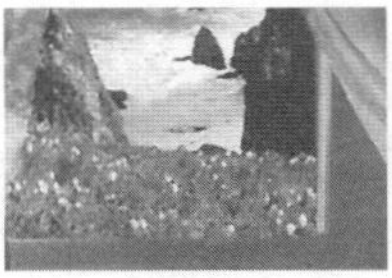

CHAPTER 2

It Takes Two to Know One

The Family System

I have longed to move away
From the hissing of the spent lie
And the old terrors' continual cry
Growing more terrible as the day
Goes over the hill into the deep sea;
I have longed to move away
From the repetition of salutes,
From ghosts in the air
And ghostly echoes on paper,
And the thunder of calls and notes.

I have longed to move away but am afraid;
Some life, yet unspent, might explode
Out of the old lie burning on the ground,
And, crackling into the air, leave me half-blind.
Neither by night's ancient fear,
The parting of hat from hair,
Pursed lips at the receiver,
Shall I fall to death's feather,
By these I would not care to die,
Half convention and half lie.

DYLAN THOMAS, *I HAVE LONGED TO MOVE AWAY*[1]

EACH OF US HAS A UNIQUE WAY that our life plays, sours, or dies. Whatever choices we make include traits and themes inherited from our families and all our ancestral ghosts. Everyone struggles with some sense of deficit from birth to death, and all of our families have contributed self-doubt in one form or another. As children we struggle with painful mysteries and, as adults, it is our responsibility to know and understand as much of the mystery as we can. We want our lives to flow beyond the wounds. I could not build a competent, passionate, creative being by stomping on the grave of my early life, by denying its difficult presence. What my deficits are, how the voids remain so persistent, and what I provide to compensate for them is essential information.

What do we know about ourselves and the family from which we came? First of all, we are never able to take for granted the existence of our alive, functioning self: our "I" must be teased out. Someone must act on us to promote our developing self and our passion for being alive. This requires parents to pay careful attention and form a dedicated relationship with us. Many parents cannot care in the way that is needed, and then we must find another guide to take their place, the earlier, the better. In several of the *voices'* lives, extended family members, an aunt, uncle, grandparent, or outside teacher stepped up. Children gained information from the new guide that they were *entitled* to be here, to know they had their own unique space. The lack of this emotional conviction or entitlement, to live and be *who you are, just the way you are,* is the beginning of a continual struggle to survive.

It has been reported that infants who are not held, do not have the capacity for emotional interactions with other people. Damage can be so profound that the infant, despite adequate physical nourishment, may wither and die. The drama of what it takes for you and me to live and grow does not escape our awareness. With the addition of multiple deflating and wrenching experiences, our lives are seriously compromised and sometimes so deadened that we become incapable of joy.

Let's focus on an extreme, those children robbed of their total sense of self. If a seriously wounded child does not emotionally die, that is, lose all his/her spiritual energy early on, then she may become an adult who dies within long before her physical body leaves this world. This child/adult lives a *death mystery.* Some children with little energy have not lived in abusive families or suffered visible wounds. Yet, emotional abandonment by the family has left them with scars and holes that no future compensation can mend. I am looking at the children who, at a very early age, have lost their alive, creative, ambitious selves. The destruction of the child's inner spirit may not be truly visible until this soul becomes an adult and now the adult cannot grab onto any persistent, creative goals, cannot find a reason for being. Thriving is marginal. The spirit is gone. When we have lived through an extended time when our music dies, some of the feelings of despair are similar.

Our destiny can be tremendously fragile. What we bring into the world — our social/psychological/biological genetic being and our unconscious self — combine to create an increased vulnerability.

The defective self and the vital creative self are powerful environments, a confusion of opposites, which expand and contract throughout our lives. My natural, psychological and biological nature as a small child was to be and act playful, funny, serious, imaginative, as well as demanding. I was an impatient and highly vocal urchin. My parents unwittingly punished this spirit. But I swam to a distant shore, kicking and stroking with the help of any aids I could grasp. Remarkably, something gave me a conviction of my rights to be who I am — an extraordinary sense of entitlement that came solely from within. But that entitlement is not my whole story.

There is one serious mystery, a deficit that has affected me and many others. How many of you have experienced the mystery of abandonment? Humans seek out relatedness to even the most foul parental caregivers to avoid being abandoned. We want to participate in a family, even knowing it can damage or kill us. We want and need to participate in a relationship, knowing we may be ignored, abused, malnourished, cast away. As adults, we will risk loss again and again, seeking bonds with significant others who support our smallest cry for attachment and love. "Many of the most *intense emotions* arise during the formation, the maintenance, the disruption, and the renewal of attachment relationships."[2]

These words of John Bowlby challenge us to a startling recognition — our spiritual being, from the time we first experienced attachment to our current love relationship — has been aware of how intense any loss would be. There is an uneasy road to attachment. We feel grief and anger deep within us when someone abandons us by living or dying.

Parents give us road maps for developing love relationships. Each of our maps suggests who and how we are to love, what emotions we may feel when we are connected with another or have lost a love relationship. This map, different for each of us, intricately proscribes how we will form and sustain future relationships. How to hold fast or give up love was one learned pattern in our family.

The way you connect and are directed to love another, what emotions you feel, how you maintain relationships, are all clues to your deepest emotional soul. Loving another requires a road map because you will follow the same paths again and again to gain your desired relationships. We can talk about the childhood psychological baggage we carry on our road to adult love. The more complete awareness we have of the road map, the better our opportunity for healthy, committed attachment. If we have not yet connected in a loving partnership, time brings us other opportunities.

In my early life my road map was pure water, a clear vision: give, do, be, act on behalf of others to guide and help. As a teenager I embroidered a large sampler that said, "Let me live in the house by the side of the road and be a friend to man." That was only one family proscription for loving attachment. Another road map defined marriage as a permanent choice without opportunities for change. The family reacted to loss by expressing anxiety and anger. What my sampler didn't say was that if you missed a beat, made a mistake, or lost a happy ending, you would be chased by powerful demons who would batter you. My divorce was a terrifying option because it appeared to be an unhappy ending. Demons showed up by the score!

Questions always arise about negative parental models, especially when love fails. We want to strike parents from the record, diminish their impact, seek ways to tell how different we are from their hated characteristics. A patient, Cary commented emphatically that his father was both physically removed by work-related travel and emotionally distanced: he had no idea "who this man was or is." Cary was angry. At a later time, he described habits, mannerisms, patterns of relationships, and values that acknowledged how much he had become his father's child. Although Cary had long ago denied that his father had any positive influence in his life, he acknowledged that this severely handicapped relationship produced in himself characteristics he had always detested in his father. Cary possessed a road map. He could not escape the power and influence of the father he had incorporated into his own being. The instructions and identification extended into all Cary's adult relationships. He recognized, dimly at first, the maddening legacy that destroyed his ability to form an intimate long-term marriage. Like his father, he behaved in a manner that opened only the smallest portion of his heart and then withdrew even that. He was impatient, dogmatic, perfectionistic, and at times cruel and sarcastic, the sins of the father revisited.

> *Not receiving any blessing from your father is an injury. . . . Robert Moore said, "If you are a young man and you're not being admired by an older man, you're being hurt." How many men have said to me, "I waited for two days with my father when he was dying, and wanted him to tell me that he loves me." What happened? "He never did. . . ." Never being welcomed into the world by older men is a wound in the chest.*[3]

Cary had played in the fields of love by building wonderful defenses to distance any loving, mature companion. Both partners fell into a cavern of angry demons so deep, nothing valuable was ever retrieved. He lived a furious and destructive personal life, but finally accepted adult responsibility.

Awareness of these patterns certainly helped Cary; he had to make a decision to change his road map. Sometimes stumbling painfully along is easier because it's all we know. What is new puts us at risk, and that is precisely where we need to be each time we love another.

We may make vows and commitments to change our agonizing patterns. But those mysteries that remain *unknown* play havoc with all our best intentions. We are rarely clueless to the chaos because harmony and well being are absent too much of the time, signaling us that something is amiss. It is then that the hard work of discovery needs to begin.

Mysteries do get solved. Intuition, our ability to perceive and understand, originates from within our partially unconscious self. It is the thoughtful, inner voice organizing those things it needs to know.

If we return to Cary's story, it was his inability to form serious attachments, a road map gained from his father, that he finally understood and challenged. Cary deserved a life that established independence and separateness from his father, *but* he could not exist without being emotionally imbedded in this relationship. It is a truth for most of us that emotional needs, sometimes very mysterious ones, keep us tied to destructive family characteristics.

When you explore your specific family of origin, the conscious and unconscious patterns of attachment become recognizable. An awareness of the tremendous influences of unconscious behavior is a major resource guiding our decisions. I chose many relationships over years that repeated my triangle, that of being left out of the tight relationship between my mother and father. Raphael, a *voice* who speaks in a later chapter, also could not enter his parent's space. There was no room for any young child. He spent many lonely hours playing alone in a basement, developing a fantasy world, while his parents worked long hours together in his father's medical office. Serious abandonment patterns existed. When Raphael and I understood the old triangles, we did not accept that our only choice was to recreate those patterns and so we moved on.

Bron is a long term friend of mine whose story gives us a beautiful window for better understanding a parent who is capable of gross abandonment. It was her mother's complete rejection of Bron which forced my friend to seek sources of love outside her family. Her mother speaks: "I would never have had you except that Doctor Smith told me to have another baby." Unlike Cary, Bron discovered mentors early on and later married a nurturing, sensitive husband, all of whom enabled her to compensate for a mother who could not love her. Her story is told within several chapters. Here are some early insights that Bron shared.

> **BRON: I always understood that my mother's story about her own life was probably true. She was the eldest, who never knew anything except raising babies. At one point there had been, I think, thirteen siblings. And she always had a baby in her hands. And her expression used to be "what did I need another baby for?" She had brought forth one baby in our family. It was a boy, which was what she wanted. The doctor across the street called her in one day and, in essence, said, "I have seen your son in this office three times in one day. You must have another baby so that it takes the heat off this child." She would say, "I would never have had you unless Dr. Smith told me to have another baby." She would tell it over and over and over again.**
>
> **As a young person growing up, I understood that very clearly: that if you had ten babies to raise, in fact, why the hell did you need another baby? There's not going to be anything new or exciting or interesting in one more baby.**
>
> **Mother went to work very early in her adolescence. When she was home, she was taking care of those siblings, and her one desire for herself, which was music, she did**

not get. Her father had told her that you have to be a very bad woman to be on the stage.

I remember my aunts calling her off me saying, "Go away. Don't do that. Leave her alone." I think one of the most telling things was that my first real doll was bought for me by the aunts. And it was quite a large doll, a foot, foot-and-a-half. I would hide that doll under my coat and take that doll to school. When I came home for lunch, I would spend most of the lunchtime bathing the baby, pretending to comb the doll's hair. And, in some way, I think I was taking care of myself. I was taking care of the baby in me.

We survive by defending ourselves from loss and abandonment. Bron had to learn to nourish herself and later to find new caring mentors and guides. Bron's mother had little conscious knowledge of her abandoning behavior; she acted on a forceful need to stop parenting her own two children. Bron's mother preferred a professional career in music. Instead, she felt coerced into raising ten brothers and sisters. Since parental disapproval closed the avenue to a career, she married at age twenty-four and later gave birth to two children. Her relationship with Bron and her younger brother incorporated old anger and disappointments. She never stopped discounting and verbally abusing Bron. Her dying breath was a statement of discontent concerning her fifty-six-year old daughter. "Why didn't you come sooner? Won't you ever get it right?"

All families have the willingness to dance a crazy way, to create loss, and all families wound their members, not with malice but with generations of dysfunction. An army of parents, grandparents, aunts, uncles, and cousins march before us. Spirits who are able to honor our soul or respect our being may be rare. In the words of Alice Miller: "The child has a primary need to be regarded and respected as the person he really is at any given time, and as the center — the central actor — in his own activity. We are speaking here of a need that is narcissistic, but nevertheless legitimate, and whose fulfillment is essential for the development of a healthy self-esteem. . . . If our parents did not experience this environment as children, they also feel deprived. Throughout their lives they are looking for what their own parents could not give them at the correct time — the presence of a person who is completely aware of them and takes them seriously, who admires and follows them."[4]

The question of different wounds for children within the same family is a familiar source of confusion among siblings. My brother, who is eight years younger than me, perceived our parents in a different way. Because he was given more freedom, he saw our mother as less domineering. Although he and I agree about some of our family history, we had very different experiences. I was the recipient of my parents' anxiety and their struggles in a difficult early marriage. By the time my brother was born family life had stabilized in a small town environment where my dad was respected. Adding more complexity, our natural responses to loss are dissimilar as well. I carry the emotions for the family.

Children want to be at one with their parents, to attach, and some parents want to believe this infant/child represents who they are, someone with whom they can bond and resonate. The infants arrive not as a blank slate but with a genetic coding — a psychological, emotional, social, and biological collection of attributes or deficiencies uniquely their own. Brough Joy, M.D., an enormously gifted teacher and writer, would say the infant is born with its own unconscious mysteries, which persist into adult life. A parents' desire to create a legacy of intuneness and children's mysteries do not always create a decent bond.

Infants and children dare to be who they are. They do this easily and intuitively until someone says no or don't do or be that. In an important sense, children reflect themselves back to the parent, creating strong feelings within the relationship. Children want empathy, they want the comfort of approval, they want non-judgmental acceptance, they want unconditional love. Rarely are children's needs for attachment and parental attention an appropriate, good fit.

A patient described her experience with three children, giving me a small perspective of the different losses that visited each sibling. The firstborn, Henry, was a colicky infant with whom the mother wished to enjoy a close relationship. The infant's constant crying and the mother's sense of failure resulted in a very stressed attachment and a withering withdrawal of love. Father sat outside the family, drawn to alcoholic addiction, and he became a ghost in the family. The mother later made desperate efforts to "right the wrong," but Henry never enjoyed a satisfying career or personal life. At age forty-two he has not formed any permanent partnerships. He has attempted many careers; none satisfy his demand to excel, and so he leaves, always looking for something different.

Henry's mother found her second child, Julie, easy to manage. Julie followed directives and patterns expected of her — nothing "unusual" occurred. When she referred to memories of her childhood, she expressed the belief that her brother was the favored child and that she was "just there." Obviously, attention and considerable energy had been consumed by Henry, the demanding, sickly first child. Righting the wrong for the firstborn created a great gap of empathic love for the middle child.

Julie involved herself with strong mentors outside the family who aided her development. Her life achievements included a career in teaching, a good marital relationship, and a family of two children who maintained closeness with each other and their parents.

The final child, Sam, was a son with several psychosomatic illnesses, including asthma. Once more, the family was taxed beyond its ability to cope. At the time of his son's birth Sam's father was unable to parent and remained completely isolated from the family. Sam defended himself by creating a substitute family. Because of many innate abilities to attract children and adults, he formed multiple relationships, many were influenced by his good humor and enjoyment of life's opportunities. His innate joy and outgoing spirit were contagious.

Although he could not receive what his father refused to give, he found compensatory male companionship, males who passed on their vitality, their interest, their love. In college he formed several relationships, which still exist today. They share tennis, football, politics, and general comradeship. He married at age twenty-seven and later became a loving, attentive father to his own sons. This gift of father/son love changed the generations of the father's neglect.

We can recognize that the father's contribution to males is different but certainly no more or less important than the gifts of the female elders to their children. I'm able in different chapters to share the legacy of four generations of women: Kay; Emily, her daughter; Emily's daughter, Cassi; as well as Emily's grandmother, now deceased. It is Emily's grandmother who supplied some of the gifts that vitalized Emily's spirit at a young age. When mothers and fathers cannot provide the soul food, another family member may step in and provide the nurturing experiences.

I met Emily a number of years ago when she was pursuing a successful business career as a dress and fabric designer. During her early years she was a professional tennis player.

Emily tells this story:

EMILY: I was born in the 1940s and my father went to war. My mother moved in with my grandmother. My mother always said I fell in love with my grandmother before I was old enough to realize it. When my father came home from the war, I must have been three or three-and-a-half. I did not want to go home with my mother. I wanted to stay with my grandmother. I was always crazy about her. She was a very strong woman and she had an enormous influence on me. She was a very hard worker. She was very kind. She was musical. She was also interested in me. I had special chemistry with my grandmother. I felt that I could count on her. I called her every day of my life. I went to all of the symphonies with her and had a complete cultural life. My home life was so traumatic because of the tennis and my grandmother buffered it.

My mother was born with a curvature of the spine and had numerous operations. She was accustomed to ill health and very sensitive to physical and mental trauma. I look upon my mother now as a fighter pilot. When she wants to do something, nothing will stop She's had all these hip surgeries and she gets up and goes to Africa alone and charges forward — enormous strength. But, I didn't see her. that when I was growing up. She was always tired. She had nine pregnancies. My father and my mother had seven children. I'm the oldest. There were six born within eight years, and then a younger brother eight years after that. Three girls and four boys.

My mother put herself on hold for forty years. She never traveled except for tennis tournaments. She just simply stayed home with her children, and later — with the trauma of my father's death — she got on an airplane and went to Paris to change her life. She did!

In 1942, my father was a doctor. He was on a ship that was bombed. The Navy brought my father back home and the Navy deposited him on my mother's doorstep. My father started practicing medicine. He also taught my brother and me to play tennis. I was five and my brother was four. My father got carried away with obsessive behaviors. We had to play every morning before school at 6:00 A.M. until school started. He would pick us up the minute school was out. We had to change in the car because he always said we didn't have a minute to lose. We would play until dark and then he would take us on house calls. We were always on the tennis court. We played every weekend. At age twelve, I was the state champion. I won about three hundred tournaments. My father was never satisfied. He pushed us all the time. I would win tournaments and he would get mad because I didn't go to the net enough. He had this personality where he became totally out of control. He could also be the kindest, sweetest, most loving, tender, sensitive person. I related to that sensitive, kind, tender side of my father. I was with him every single day of my life and so when he was kind, I remembered.

My father was a strong role model in that he was dedicated to something. I grew up learning how to be dedicated. I mean I am very disciplined. I am like my father — that sensitive side, that loving humor. But, also, if I let myself go, I could be too fanatical.

> **For years, I did nothing but play tennis. I was always winning for my father. I was not motivated to be the world's greatest tennis player. I felt inadequate. I didn't feel that he didn't love me. I felt that I disappointed him. The thing that I find most fascinating is that my father was abusive. This wasn't a private abuse. He was out in front of everyone at the country club, screaming at us and hitting balls at us.**

Emily shares the pain created by her father's patriarchal proscriptions for her identity. The abusive, demanding, controlling father she experienced as a child was later understood as a father who returned from the war with an untreated obsessive mental illness. Her mother Kay was seen as a buffer to her father's obsessive illness, as well as a remarkable caretaker of an ill husband and seven children. Kay was unable to prevent the damage her husband's obsessive control had on Emily's and Bob's tennis careers. Kay did attend most games in an effort to soften the critical blows.

There are ways we recognize and understand the legacy of our primary caregivers. Sometimes therapy is needed to do this. Understanding parents enables us to better know our self because it takes two to know one. Even weak parents have powerful legacies. Parental influences are scattered over our mental landscape. Unconsciously we store them within our minds and they will remain mainly untouched unless we can uncover a new reality, with new perceptions replacing the original images. Emily discovered her father's illness as a prelude to emotional abuse. As an adult Bron discovered her mother's history of disappointment, which led to the emotional abandonment of both siblings.

Perhaps your life as a child creates a perfect coloring book to fill in portraits of your mother and dad and to create some fantasy portraits and myths as well. This perception of your parents becomes your truth, a seemingly incontrovertible belief. The colors may be fixed, rigid, unaltered by time. One image of my parents was an understanding that they were devoted to each other but not responsive to my childhood needs. It was difficult to soothe myself, to experience calmness, because my parents could not teach me this. Self-soothing came to me much later as an adult but only after years of pain and anxiety. In this portrait, I was accurate about the legacy.

Must you respond only to these parental identifications? Do your adult actions and choices depend only on the traits and deficits you have learned? The answer to this question is no.

You are in the middle of your movie: you *cannot* rewrite the earliest scenes of your life or change the original picture of who you were at birth. You did respond to early parental action, and will use some of these old childhood identifications during your entire life. But we can and do change important ways of acting and being.

I identified with my mother's perfectionism, everything always in its place. My mother was born late, well after four brothers. She was the little princess, treated like a doll, responsible for being the perfect child. Her father died when she was seven. My mother's mother judged every act, at the same time keeping her only daughter tightly emotionally attached. Because only two women existed in the household, my grandmother insisted that my mother sleep in her bedroom, allowing no separation or appropriate boundaries. The excuse was safety. When I gave birth to twins later in life, my parenting was no doubt influenced by what I'd witnessed early in my life. I established from the beginning that each was an independent child with a distinct and unique personality. I hoped they would hear their own music.

There is a saving grace. You and I are not only what our parents created. We bring to our life our own unique makeup, a soul that is different from theirs. We change the tapestry of our life when we seek new mentors, guides, and friends who support our true spirit. We change our tapestry when we exert every intention to hear our inner voice, to know what is our unknown mystery.

WE HAVE A SPACE WE CAN ENTER, ONE THAT PROVIDES AN ENLIGHTENED PERCEPTION OF OUR ORIGINAL FAMILY: PROVIDES KNOWLEDGE OF OUR DEFICIT-RIDDEN SELF AND OUR SHAMED PERSON: PROVIDES GRIEF AND OUR COMPASSION FOR ALL THE WOUNDS AND ALL THE LOSSES (THAT IS CALLED SELF-SOOTHING): PROVIDES NON-JUDGMENTAL AIR TO BREATHE: PROVIDES RESOURCES TO EXPRESS OUR EMOTIONS: AND FINALLY PROVIDES A CHOSEN DESTINY IN WHICH WE DO NOT NEED TO FAIL AGAIN AND AGAIN.

The new space can provide hope, grace, and unconditional love. Our effort as adults to know and understand the ghosts, the unconscious demons, and images of all who came before us — to know where they stand — is powerful material if we are to create a life of greater choice and inviolable freedom. At the deepest level we can create a loving spiritual acceptance of ourselves and the others. We provide a re-enchantment of our lost spirit.

The journey to achieve this space is lifelong. We do this in small parts and on a daily basis. We do this alone and in the presence of guides, therapists, mentors, and friends. If we add the smallest pieces of understanding to our unique mystery, we have enriched our soul, amended our life.

Notes to Chapter 2

1. Dylan Thomas, *The Collected Poems of Dylan Thomas* (New York: James Laughlin, 1952), p. 73.
2. John Bowlby, *Loss, Sadness, and Depression* (New York: (Basic Books Inc./Harper, 1980), p. 40.
3. Robert Bly, *Iron John* (Toronto: Vintage Books and Random House of Canada, 1990), pp. 31–32. The "Robert Moore" mentioned in the quotation is author of the book, *King Warrior Magician Lover.*
4. Alice Miller, *The Drama of the Gifted Child* (New York: Basic Books, Inc., 1981), p. 7.

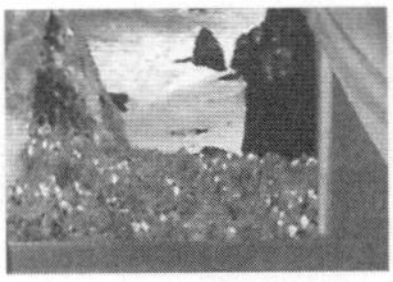

CHAPTER 3

Boundaries and Entitlement

We cannot hope to find a view of man that will be independent of the context in which we find ourselves, the purpose we follow, the assumptions we make. Sometimes, likewise, it will be necessary to see (our) behavior — as the product of unconstrained will for we are truly free, even in situations of extreme coercion.

ALLEN WHEELIS[1]

DURING MY INFANCY AND CHILDHOOD my mother established confusing boundaries. The physical, mental, and emotional space between us was distorted because our relationship seesawed between little involvement by her and an overkill of attention in which my own decisions were wrestled from me. My mother's mother overprotected her only daughter, and this became increasingly severe at age seven when my grandfather died. My grandmother's guidance was an overwrought protection of her only daughter in a family of four, much older sons. Until my mother married at age seventeen, all her decisions were dominated by my determined grandmother who believed control of her children would keep everyone from harm's way.

My mother was given the least freedom to be herself. Her parenting of me was a reflection of her own diminished boundaries and a conflicted ideal about giving me freedom to grow. As a result, my own efforts to maintain consistent boundaries were a struggle until I reached my middle years. The pathway of mangled boundaries was fixed, I suspect, before I knew the difference between my mother and myself.

There is so much the mother provides that is unconscious as she holds, speaks to, and goes about necessary tasks for her infant and, later, young child. What appears to be unimportant mutual adaptation on the part of the child and the mother figure, is in reality an opportunity to discover clues concerning how we, as adults, form *intimate relationships.* Throughout many years I needed to know someone waited in the wings to rescue me if my partnership failed. I finally understood an important clue, revealed to me when I began to examine the impact of my parent's triangle, the tight interactions between them, which excluded me from feeling secure. To feel safe I required a "backup person" who I was sure loved me.

We learn a great deal from infants who are removed from parents, often through death, especially in war-torn countries in Eastern Europe. These infants have such limited touching and care that their emotional, intellectual, and even physical development is impaired. Children in Romanian orphanages are reported to be much smaller in growth than would be expected under normal conditions. Stunted growth is a quantifiable measurement but later studies will be done to understand more about the emotional consequences of being abandoned as an infant. What we can expect is that many of these untouched children will be emotionally and spiritually isolated and deadened, distanced from intimate relationships.

Even children born into a stable family are forever adapting to the space provided by parents as the family limits or continually stretches itself to accommodate new members. The family is like a giant rubber band shrinking and stretching to exclude and include all its members. This can be observed clearly when two families blend; some children are left out and others are welcomed. At its best, all children would fit and be included in their own unique way, but family life doesn't provide many healthy rubber bands. Families that tolerate, accept, and even nurture the differences that make each child unique, each born with its own mystery, are rare.

Boundaries between people refer to not only the physical space but, most importantly, emotional and mental distance. Each of us has a different comfort level concerning how close we are willing to be to another. In my twenties I needed physical and emotional distance from my parents and made a difficult decision to move from the East coast to California, creating a large space between us. If I had remained near them, our contact would have been daily, with inclusion of strong emotional influences from my mother. I had to leave, knowing I needed space to develop my own voice, to develop my personality, different from hers.

If you return to earliest memories, you may recall events that were crucial to your sense of failed or unclear boundaries. What clues indicate failure? The person who speaks for another; the family member who opens your mail or listens when you speak on the telephone; the person who tells you what to feel, what to do; the person who completes your sentence, tells your stories, acts on your behalf, stands in your face, lives your life.

Each of us is entitled to establish our own rules, to say, don't cross this line. When we experience deep and consistent wrenching pain, it may signal a penetrating intrusion of our emotional, mental, or physical space, our boundaries violated.

IF YOU DO NOT PARTICIPATE IN THE ADULT RULES OF YOUR RELATIONSHIPS, THEN RESTRUCTURING DAMAGED BOUNDARIES IS IMPOSSIBLE.

Within many families are over-involved members — familial relations that are enmeshed. The child who must hold mother's apron all day as she goes about her tasks is a powerful symbol of enmeshment. Heather, a friend of mine, speaks about a family system so entwined that no one escaped unharmed. She is now sixty-five years old. This is a part of her story. It was her sister as a small child who was instructed to hold mother's apron, and as an adult she now symbolically holds Heather's, creating tremendous pain as boundaries continually crumble between them.

HEATHER: I have in my lifetime, going back to adolescence, had to suppress feelings due to family situations and health problems. My father had a heart attack. I was thrown into the workforce without being able to graduate from business school.

Feelings were not to be shown in my family. You were to withstand things, be brave, have courage. You were to walk straight, shoulders back, and personify someone who could handle the situation. This was very evident when my father had his massive heart attack. We were not to go into the room and show feelings. I found trouble turning it on and turning it off. I was suppressed for so long. When I did get out of the suppressed mode, I was a basket case. I would cry, and cry, and cry, and get exhausted with it.

Now you'll have to stay in town, and have courage and carry on because you've got the responsibility of this family. That would be hard for one at any age. That wasn't too easy in your late teens and early twenties. Especially when you're just starting out in the business world, starting your own career. I tried different things to work around it.

I first thought it was a temporary issue. However, as time went by, and even years went by — after I made some physical changes, moving to another state, taking another job, and so forth — I thought I would be able to escape it, get away from it, go into a different life pattern. But as I moved, so did they. One always followed. If it wasn't the sister, it was the mother, or whatever, and then in the interim the father passed away.

I did date people, but I found myself suppressing the sensitivity of it. I would draw a line. Knowing what the situation was with the family, I could not bring myself to disregard the family obligations, or to drop everything and just go my own way, have my own life.

We were raised that you don't forget family. We were raised that family was family. I look back on it now, and I find it quite unbelievable. Everyone's problem was everyone's problem. Anyone who had a problem of a serious nature became an extended family problem. Then, someone from the family was summoned to rescue the victim. But, in my case, I — being the baby of the family — got all the trickled-down emotions and the trickled-down stress, the trickled-down suppression. I mean it trickled right down to the baby, me.

When you are suddenly responsible for the checkbook and the survival for three people plus yourself, there's no way you would miss work. You had to go to work sick,

> **unless you were in the hospital, because you brought home the bacon. You were the survivor.**
>
> **I wouldn't take my own stand. I went along with the system, dysfunctional as it may have been. I guess I was too young to understand identifications and what was involved. I was just doing what had to be done. I was working and I was doing so many other things that I was in a three-ring circus. Even if I tried to get away from it, I could never. You cannot run away from a problem, no matter how far you go.**
>
> **Now, other people don't like the way I stand in my own shoes because I have taken on a new persona, a new identity. Some people, even in my own family, think that I'm strange or that I am not like I used to be, or not as sensitive. Now I have set my priorities, where before I was following everybody else's priorities and everybody else's wants and desires. Now that I have set my own agenda, it does not go down too well with the others.**

There is a large, extended family judging Heather's decisions to separate herself emotionally and live according to her own needs and desires. In this family, mother and father have died and Heather, age sixty-five, has become a caretaker of her ill sister, age seventy. The old parental identification of taking care of family still persists, as does the pain of Heather's inability to live a physically separate existence. Heather has made some independent decisions, but both women are enraged that they must live in one house and at times have been unable to find any acceptable means of creating boundaries. Emotionally and financially, they are tied together, even though Heather takes charge of her own life as much as she can. Heather is emotionally imbedded in her sister's life and feels responsible for her well being. The sisters live with their own, separate locked doors and cupboards in an effort to preserve their own boundaries and claim something as their own.

Family affiliations and personal relationships are not cast in concrete: that means we can reclaim our own boundaries and establish workable limits. Freedom doesn't imply a license for another person to intrude upon or to squash our authentic space, so we are the final arbitrator of our boundary. I am acknowledging that we cannot control the behavior of others, their intrusion, or their exclusion. Heather's sister refuses to leave the family home and would need to be legally evicted, which is an impossible emotional task; however, Heather recently discovered another option.

What we require to live comfortably, what is our "must be" is fortunately within our domain. When our rules are unacceptable to others, we can make a choice to withdraw from those relationships. There are as many stages of withdrawal as there are of attachment. Withdrawing entirely from a relationship may not be our best choice; we may prefer to create some distance instead. Setting limits and maintaining our balance are difficult tasks, always waiting for us. We set limits only to find something has occurred that requires further action to regain a balance.

There is a boundary exercise I have found helpful. Take several minutes for quiet reflection or meditation and think of the word "distance." When you are sharply focused on this thought, you will become intuitively aware of the best boundary at this time. "Distance" can mean making a decision about distancing yourself, or it can mean making a decision to take actions that move you closer to another. Step up or step back. Your inner voice may know what is appropriate even when the choices are extremely difficult. A patient of mine mentioned that the child-like part of himself frequently responded with anxious emotions to important events. When he learned to create some distance, the mature adult part of him was able to be present and respond more appropriately. He would step back and stop participating for a brief time. This gave him a more objective, intuitive perception, one devoid of gut level, emotional response. This small shift changed his relationship with everyone in his life.

I'll share a similar experience. On a recent trip, I had to negotiate with my spouse concerning the time spent with family members versus a visit I wished to share alone with a college roommate. I could have obliterated my boundary by accepting pressure to forego the visit with my friend. Although I was angry, I stepped back and reflected on the word "distance," as we've just discussed. As a compromise my husband and I negotiated the comfort level of visiting for shorter periods with everyone. Both of us adapted to our separate and individual needs. At a different moment in time there might have been a priority for me to make a more self-centered choice, that is, no compromise.

My inner voice spoke intuitively. My emotional, angry self was totally removed from the intuitive response I received. I want to emphasize an important distinction: Emotions and intuition are different functions, often mistaken for each other. Emotion represents a judgment, a feeling that something should be a specific way. Intuition is an inner path of perceiving the world, a thinking function, which usually takes in a big picture. When we feel something strongly we may believe it's our intuition, but intuition is *not a feeling function.* Intuition is an inner knowing, mental clarity, originating through our unconscious access to a great variety of information.

Two more aspects of relationships and boundaries need to be considered. Interdependency and dependency are directly involved with all the rules of relationship. When you are interdependent you do not rely on another as though your entire survival is dependent on that person. Your perspective is that you are a whole being. You recognize that your human needs include the caring, attention, warmth, and love of others. Because you need others in your life, you form interdependent relationships, that is, fully acknowledging the give and take of a fulfilling association. Do you have the knowledge that you can interact as a strong, autonomous self with another equally whole person? If the answer is yes, then you are responding as a partner in an interdependent relationship. Dependency is not wholeness; it is merging with another to gain a sense of being a complete person. One plus one equals one.

But another dimension and complication is present. Your ability to participate in a joyous relationship is predicated on knowing where your "I" stops and the "WE" begins. The autonomous "I" and the integrated "WE" are both necessary parts of the self, to be continually balanced. Frequently the need for "WE" activity is dissimilar in partners.

Many of us have been carefully taught that being autonomous is selfish. Have you ever been thrown into a wall of negativity and betrayal, fed by voices that say your actions as a separate, functioning "I" are selfish and wrong? That was the message Heather received from her family. Your soul is your own and when you make decisions to nurture and protect it, you are making a choice that is self-centered and healthy. In fact, this kind of decision, in the long run, is generous, since it is through our soul that we make our greatest contribution.

When we form alliances with people who are very different from ourselves, fear of intimacy may arise. What is the effect of uniquely different personalities attempting to form an interdependent relationship? Can opposites complement each other?

There is an initial fascination with people who are very different from ourselves, but this may fade rapidly. The other person can quickly become an opposer to our values, beliefs, needs. We fear confrontation or being overwhelmed. We struggle to maintain our own integrity and yet allow this stranger, who is a different thinking/feeling person, to become part of our world. That is a serious challenge.

I believe opposites can be complementary. We can participate both as a separate self and as an opposite, complementary part of another person. "Rejoicing in the opposites means pushing the opposites apart with our imaginations so as to create space, and then enjoying the fantastic music coming from each side."[2]

Opposites do need an abundance of space to play. Bron kept herself removed from her mother so that she would know what was truly her own gift. Later, Raphael will speak about the space he created to survive his relationship with a demanding, overbearing father. Each of us can best appreciate the gifts of another when we feel safe that we will not be buried by them.

The space we create as an adult functions best when separate from our parents' domain. The road we take when we enter our private space will be different from our parents'. We cannot go home again on a permanent basis and maintain our integrity. Adult boundaries require separate space.

One patient shared a very rich dream relating to the development of his own world: He was in his mother's house, needing to protect a domesticated, big, old, and beautiful cat. Outside the house, which covered many acres of farmland, were feral cats — wild, wild cats — that threatened the domesticated mother cat. My patient wanted to blow up the wild cats even though he was put off by the idea of hurting them. Yet, he needed to get rid of them because they endangered the household cat. There was a final image: the patient noted that a tall building had appeared on the land; its appearance was strange and curious, he thought, because this building did not belong on this property.

In our work together we explored the many levels of interpretation in this dream. I want to punctuate just a few: The tall building was his manhood and his male spirit self, which could not exist or develop in his mother's space — he knew the tall building was "on the wrong property." As long as he protected the mother cat — a symbol of female, domesticated values, emotions, beliefs and perceptions — he could not partake of his own identification. He had no space to maintain his true self — his "wild" self.

He wanted to blow up his Wild Man, or the parts he had "thrown away": the passionate, vital, assertive, creative male nature as symbolized by the feral cats. He had abandoned these qualities but they always came back, as did the feral cats in the dream. "The Wild Man's qualities, among them love of spontaneity, association with wilderness, honoring of grief, and respect for riskiness frightens many people. Some men, as soon as they receive the first impulses to riskiness and recognize its link with what we've called the Wild Man, become frightened, stop all wildness, and recommend timidity and collective behavior to others."[3]

Some part of my patient's male spirit saw that these wild qualities needed to exist even if they completely endangered the domestic values. In fact, he understood he would need to confront his mother's values and beliefs in order to develop his own worthy self. He could not be merged with the domestic cat. He must separate. The tall building that is his own male identity, would need to be built on his own land, separate from his mother and his father.

Returning to the "domesticated" home, to the rigid systems of our parents, can restrict all that is valuable and unique within our spirit, telling it not to evolve. This return is not simply a physical step to live in a parent's home. It is reentering the values, beliefs, goals, and proscriptions that are thrust upon us, even by our loving parents. "Our work then as men and women is not only to free ourselves from family cages and collective mind sets, but to release transcendent beings from imprisonment and trance. That's what the story says in the end."[4]

Entitlement is an important element of boundaries. Two opposite energies are at work here: in most families entitlement is based on a play between abundance and scarcity.

Let's first take a look at the energy of scarcity. When experiences and feelings assault the self-esteem of family members, large holes develop and the core self is punctured with deficit, like old Swiss cheese. As family members withhold attention, love, kindness, empathy, and support, a mood is created. Family members withdraw from one another. Soon there is a sense of stinginess, pungent and sharp, very different in feeling from the expansive, loving acts of generosity. The young, still developing self, cannot experience feelings of gratitude for the love and caring that are so seriously missing. Ultimately, there is a substantial lack of generosity, to which all the family members may be exposed, and like a contagious disease it spreads from one to another. The reality that forms with such an environment is that there is never enough to satisfy these needs of this family. The symbols of dissatisfaction can be perceived as material things — clothes, a home, trips, cars, entertainment — but the underlying void is love and empathy. Our own behaviors within this environment, which lack the spirit of giving, are founded most frequently in an early failure of parental generosity. The parent is emotionally stingy and the child's worldview of scarcity includes feelings of envy and jealousy, or perceptions that others have more of what he or she desires. The children of the stingy parents believe they do not deserve nor can get what they desire. Often this is an unconscious pattern. Perhaps you have been unable to connect the origin of envy as it relates to scarcity. Both begin with your emotional malnourishment, sometimes expressed as being "starved for love." The difficulty for us in perceiving this malnourishment may be that there has never been any direct abuse. There is in its place perhaps, an attitude of neglect, a spectacular lack of interest, or even emotional intimidation. The child cast into such a void is just as vulnerable to scarcity as a child who is physically beaten or even sexually abused. The parent maintains a remarkably distanced boundary, leaving the child with only its self as emotional support. Self-soothing is incredibly difficult for a child.

At the other end of the spectrum is abundance and generosity of spirit: a reflection that the world contains enough for each and every family member to be fulfilled. In some families we are educated and given an unalterable trust that our spirit will be loved. We feel entitled. It is not to say that our young ego is without any deficit or longing for more empathic loving, but we can experience what is *plentiful.* We experience a profound trust in our own being and from this reality, we construct our own belief and trust in abundance. We reach out to the world with its marvelous generosity and we happily give this same abundance to others.

The boundaries of abundance are close but not intrusive; they are loving, nourishing, and soothing. The parents maintain appropriate closeness to the child, neither hovering like a mother hen herding her brood or a bird of prey waiting to pounce, or so removed that the child feels a cold presence —

distanced and unfeeling. In a family of scarcity the child walks around like an intruder on an alien planet. Imagine being chilled to the bone. In scarcity, boundaries are distant, uncomplimentary, and certainly not affectionate. In abundance the child feels the presence of others in a natural, comfortable, loving manner. Like a cat sitting in the sun, we feel a radiance of warmth.

Are you an alchemist who can transform silver to gold, scarcity to abundance? I believe scarcity is an issue of the core self, lodged deep within our soul and difficult to change. It is a cold wind that blows through our heart. However, the heartiest ambition to reconstruct a new view of abundance in our life goes a long way to effectively change the scarcity perception of the world. The desire to be generous becomes one act followed by another and then another. Abundance follows you and you become the first recipient of a new generosity. Where once our music stopped, now we can experience a re-enchantment of our vital spirit.

Within our unconscious self are memories of early experiences that are capable of enhancing self-worth or positive self-knowledge, or perhaps at least some small memories of abundant events. If we can access the positive memory, our perception of what we inherited changes. Working with our dreams, fantasies, guided images, and different forms of therapy, memories surface that are both painful and positive. For some, the wounds of the child were so miserable that everything is denied or repressed — the good acts, the emotionally healthy events, the joy of a happy day, along with the damaging experiences. Everything gets lumped together and lost to memory. Remembering some moments of grace and joy, remembering who you are can be a powerful tool for transcending your wounds. When we begin to live healthy moments of generosity we can unconditionally love ourselves. If you cannot remember any past experiences of love and abundance, then create them in your present life and they will bring generosity to your otherwise scarce or barren tapestry. Amy's story, which I'll tell soon, illustrates an enormous effort and enormous success . . . transforming a legacy of scarcity to abundance.

Before telling Amy's story, I want to share a personal event. Many years after leaving home I returned for a brief visit in the fall. It was one of those incredible New England shows of color — gold, red, persimmon orange, and green. The leaves on the ground smelled faintly of burning maple syrup. I walked the streets in early morning as lights began to brighten kitchens and smoke curled from chimneys. A dog howled. A brown and white cow tied to a tree in a side yard reminded me of how rural this small college town was. I scuffed along the long street of historical homes (smelling the dank mysterious mixture of odors), my feet pushing maple leaves just as I had done years ago. The fallen leaves scrunched under my feet. Suddenly I remembered the joy of early fall, leaves burning, pumpkins, cakes, apples, humor . . . that was it. Humor, the saving grace. When I entered my parent's house with red and yellow bittersweet plants in hand, a special smell of baking cake filled the hall. My mother and I laughed about the fallen orange cake incident so many years ago, the fallen cake that looked like a small pancake. I was happy to be in my mother's kitchen, grateful for a morning of unsurpassed beauty, walking once again with joy as the color and frost touched my deepest heart. My childhood memories and the remains of the day melded. Peace was restored. I will remember that day always.

Re-enchanting our spirit, by relinquishing memories of painful or difficult periods of our lives, requires a major drive . . . a belief and trust in the process. We act on what we believe. If we believe we can be generous, we will act generously. Forgiving my mother began with acts of mutual generosity on that frosty day in October... an orange cake, a handful of bittersweet.

But let's return to my friend Amy. She and I met many years ago. She was a most attractive, talented but struggling artist. I sensed a deep well of pain and yet a determination to succeed. And succeed she did, although there were many dark tunnels along the way. Her creativity is drawn from the depths of an emotionally malnourished child. Amy's poignant story is a dramatic example of poor boundaries, abuse, inconsistent expectations unfairly visited on one sibling, and Amy's resulting belief that she didn't deserve to be loved, nor was she entitled to live abundantly.

> **AMY: My sister would torture me. When I would walk into the house she would turn off all the lights, shove me in, and say, "Ha, ha, find the light." She would take a sweater, swing it around until the buttons hurt me. As they hurt me, I would be screaming, and she would keep hitting me with them. But, during the same years she would tell me wonderful stories. So, I would want the stories, and I would put up with the abuse.**
>
> **I was basically the scapegoat of the family. I had no witness. I was the baby and was always seen as too emotional. I think, in some ways, I acted out the anger and emotion of the whole family. They were always in control. Their intellect always got them through. I loved music and art. My mother was smart enough to get me involved in piano lessons, singing, and art lessons. Art really became the pipeline to my sanity.**
>
> **I think my mother knew that I was different but she didn't know quite how to cope. If I was messy, instead of**

sitting with me and teaching me how to clean up my room, she would beat me up and throw all my clothes, all my stuff in the middle of the room, scream and say "clean it up." I'm sure I acted out my anger by being messy. If I would do ten good things, and one thing that wasn't good, she would focus on, "Oh, you'll always be selfish."

I was abused by my father in the sense that he didn't protect me from my mother. My father came home every day. I'm sure he must have heard me screaming when my mother would come in and beat me up. He never did a thing. He never said, "Don't do that."

I was really terrified most of my childhood. I used my intellect, I remember when I got my first 99, it was like the world had come to an end for my mother. She needed 100 percent. I was student body president in high school and all of that, but on another level it was like I had to perform because the core inside of me was rotten.

In order to be in that family, I had to behave. I wasn't allowed to be emotional. I wasn't allowed to yell or misbehave. I wasn't allowed to be messy. They preferred me to be invisible, but when I was present, I had to perform, play the piano, look pretty, or say funny things. They would laugh at my jokes because I had a nice sense of humor. None of the dark side was ever accepted. I also felt, in some way, that there was a double message from my mother — don't be too smart, or too confident, or too successful, nobody will love you. That was a very important message.

You have to understand. I adored my brother, my sister, my mother, and my father. In other words, you know, you always love the perpetrator because there's good stuff you're getting as well. So, you put up with the bad stuff in order to get the good stuff. This has been the story of my

life and my relationships. I would sustain a certain amount of abuse or dysfunctional behavior on the part of men to get the good stuff. I think I've been repeating that pattern.

Speaking of her husband: I wasn't really accepted. As long as I put on a happy face and did it his way, it was wonderful. I was pretty unhappy the first year. There was a part of me that knew there was a whole side of me that he really couldn't accept. Maybe, if I had a more functional adult inside instead of that needy little girl, I would have learned how to stand up to him. But, basically he was a patriarch and I was submissive. During the marriage, I was terrified that he would yell. I did everything I could so that he wouldn't. But there's always that fear.

As we share Amy's wrenching story, she clarifies the wounds perpetuated by a family where very little fair balance existed. The entire family conspired in the abuse; the females, mother and sister, taking active roles; the males, father and brother, being silent witnesses. Amy's mother projected on Amy her own parental proscriptions, unhappiness and expectations . . . expectations to be a pretty performer, to be an unemotional person, or worst of all, to be invisible. All of these combined to wipe out Amy's needs, wipe out parts of Amy's soul. For thirty years she lost boundaries and entitlement to be herself, but found her own restoration of her true spirit in the middle of her life.

Amy slowly built new patterns within her personal and professional life. She discovered a new creativity by moving to a city more receptive to her artistic work. That step alone began a series of changes. She needed courage to move to a new city and she gained this support from several spiritual and therapeutic experiences. Her talent as an artist, thinker, and writer were now more accepted and appreciated. During this same time she established a nurturing relationship with a supportive male. Amy has finally found some of the lost parts of herself.

Some of her older paintings reflect her chaos and turmoil, busy images crowded onto one canvas. Her restored spirit is illuminated now in the peaceful images of her latest works of art. The spaces on canvas symbolically reflect more appropriate personal boundaries. The images are not competing, falling all over each other: rather, there is space for each entity to exist in color, beauty, and mystery.

"The most neatly tended suburban house can contain a jungle. The one who appears to the world as the 'good sibling,' meeting all outward criteria of health, may be the worst exploited and the most vulnerable."[5] The so-called bad child as well as the good child expect to hold the family together, each believing they can focus the family on themselves. The bad child is often painfully unentitled and is burdened with debts to be what everyone else wants. Amy had to be unemotional. Amy had to perform as well as disappear on cue. In her childhood, Amy believed she was the bad one. Or at other times, the good one, holding the family together. Strangely enough she was able to use the parts of her mother that loved art and culture to build major themes and resources to gain a sense of self and to hear her music. Later I will tell you a story, relating to Amy's restoration, which brought her beyond an ordinary experience to a spiritual path and the richer material in her life.

Amy, Heather, and I stand always in a context with all our relations. We stand sometimes in pain and confusion about the past and present. We are known by our connections — Amy and her mother, Heather and her sister, my mother and me. It takes two to know one.

Many of us are never fully satisfied with the journey of our spirit and it frequently lacks something, some oppressive void forms, some ghost speaks to us in the night, whispers in our ear, does not allow us to rest in peace.

Secretly, I thirst for acceptance, for a belief that I am wonderful just the way I am, for attachments that I can trust, for connections with those who will not judge me.

Jan Oxenberg made a documentary film of mother, daughter, and grandmother relationships. She said, "Maybe Mother Teresa's mother was perfectly satisfied with her daughter."[6] Probably not, for even saints have ghosts who call to them in the night.

Notes to Chapter 3

1. Allen Wheelis, *The Quest for Identity* (New York: W.W. Norton & Co., 1958), p. 96.
2. Robert Bly, *Iron John* (Toronto: Vintage Books and Random House of Canada,1990), p. 175.
3. Ibid., p. 226.
4. Ibid., p. 233.
5. Ivan Boszormenyi-Nagy, M.D. and David N. Ulrich, Ph.D. in *Handbook of Family Therapy,* eds. Alan S. Gurman and David P. Kniskern (New York: Brunner/Mazell, 1981), p. 160.
6. Jan Oxenberg, as stated on *All Things Considered,* National Public Radio.

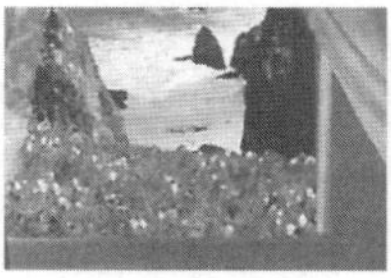

CHAPTER 4

The Spirit Self

What Is Our Essence and True Design?

Every Individual has two courses open to him and every individual, either one way or another, follows both of them. In his ordinary day every man lives by the pleasure and reality principles: He is the man of work and love. But no man is excluded from participating in the tragic dimensions of life. There will be periods, or at least moments, in the life of every man when he becomes aware, even if only dimly, of a yearning that does not relate to the attainment of the pleasurable wishes but to the compelling urge to realize the deep-rooted design of his nuclear self.

HEINZ KOHUT[1]

ON AN ORDINARY DAY I THINK ABOUT work and love, what I am doing, how much it satisfies me, would my life be happier if. . . ? I wonder if my spirit can maintain a creative life? Will tomorrow fulfill a deeper purpose, a longing on my part to capture the essence of my richer self? Those thoughts occur to me in small and yet sometimes obtrusive ways. I know I live with deficits, voids that exist simultaneously with my creativity and passion, voids that can shut down my music. This thought repeats in my mind, I will need to accept partial healing of my original wounds, which have been my mystery since birth. When healing fails, it fails badly, as it did recently when a talented author committed suicide at the height of his creativity. "Man is born broken. He lives by mending."[2]

To create, regain and maintain a healthy, vibrant self has been a lifelong effort on my part. I needed some help to guide my understanding of why I believed some aspects of myself were left unsatisfied and what if anything had really *failed,* perhaps since birth. I know I am pushed from within to satisfy my goals, ambitions, and ideals. Any time I perceive that I have failed in either part I feel guilt, shame, and a profound lack of worth. When it's at its worst I know that my failed expectations about what I need to achieve can kill me. I am a cancer survivor who has experienced firsthand how the relationship of our minds and bodies affect wellness.

I will share some historical information about the way ambition and ideals develop and work. We acquire aims and ambitions in our earliest years and their development is dependent on our experiences with parents, who we first recognize and want to please. Aims to accomplish something are probably formed in the second year of life when we understand this is me. We acquire our early original motivation to choose and act on a goal from our mother or a caregiver, always with a wish to gain her love and acceptance. As small childen, these ambitions to achieve, to exhibit our skills, are obviously little and limited, but don't underestimate their importance. We test other people, seeking their approval of our accomplishments, at the very beginning of our efforts to achieve success. Do you remember bringing home your first drawings or papers from school? Can you hear your mother saying "it's not neat, you did not give the right answers." Or, worst of all, do you remember being sent away hastily because she was too busy to respond at all? Though you may not have known it your ambition was temporarily injured and undermined.

Without empathetic, supportive parents we are disabled from achieving goals until we can acquire new sources, new teachers to encourage our ambition. Bron and I relied heavily on new mentors. Bron, in seventh grade, was brought under the wings of a caring, inspiring, principal/teacher. I found my first mentors in a small private high school, some were older peers, and others were teachers. I especially recall a biology teacher who praised my dissection of a frog. My mother was overjoyed because she assumed I'd become a doctor. I felt wonderful for a short time because a career in medicine was valued by my parents, and that meant they valued me. I married two physicians, and much later, I became a Ph.D. . . . There are no accidents!

What can I say about the second part, the ideals? From my vantage point, this is especially important. All through life we have a vision of many ideals. Planted ahead on a mountain path is a flag, a potential, an ideal. Think of your own ideals. What are they? Ideals are those standards you consider worthy, those things you value. They represent the principles that are most desirable, no matter what our ambition. In my life, ideals I value are honesty, ethical behavior, and fairness; another of my ideals is that I want my relationships with others to be totally without conflict, regardless of the challenge. One final ideal that I demanded of myself was to be the best I could be in all my career goals, and all my personal choices.

What we value can contain images of excellence, if not perfection. We must always perform to a given standard, no matter what the circumstance allows. It is our ego sometimes saying "I don't want to be OK with this; I want to be perfect." Most high achievers and creative people recognize the need to be perfect or, at least, outstanding.

Ideals are part of our *idealized self*, which is a picture of who we want to be. We are never far-removed from shame or guilt as we struggle to measure up, to fulfill the idealized self we believe is necessary, even demanded by our own ego. If we can't be this person, we may say goodbye to peace and well-being. During my life I sculpted on marble using an air hammer. It's a powerful tool to create rough cuts on hard stone. After the first process of hammering the initial form, file and sandpaper are used to refine the sculpture. During my early years I used a metal air hammer on my fragile spirit. I hammered and hammered, measuring up to overwhelming expectations. My idealized self required enormous efforts to be continually excellent. When I hammered in the wrong direction, the stone fragmented leaving only small pieces of a once beautiful form. That same destruction is exactly what happened to me for a long time. I stopped using the air hammer on my spirit; fine sandpaper was finally enough.

"*Ideals are guides, not gods.* If they become gods, they stifle man's playful creativeness."[3] If the ideal is a god, you are very likely living with perfectionism, those deadly proscriptions without *flexibility* or *acceptance of disappointment.* Ideals are not a destination; they are only a map, some directions given during our long journey. If our playful creative self is shut down by godlike ideals, re-enchantment of our spirit is nearly impossible.

My mother and father were both active in building ideals. They spoke frequently about principles of behavior and accomplishments they admired. My parents had a friend who was a local judge. I remember how much they appreciated his personal ideals, as well as the standards he ruled on daily in his court. More awareness of what I had accepted from my parents surfaced in my early adulthood. There were always multiple ideals floating near me: trust, honesty, perfect habits, brother's keeper, cleanliness, order, work, a standard of aesthetics, and so on. For many years, I could barely keep up with my standards of excellence.

My family had pockets of acceptable chaos. The metaphor and reality were secret, messy drawers of paper in an antique piece of furniture called a secretary desk. My own obsessive perfection required a continual effort to amend and order my surroundings. No messy drawers! Two things were created when I became the mother of twins; one was fatigue, accompanied by too little time to accomplish my own playful experiences. The second was an annoying anxiety when I could not maintain a standard of order, impossible to fulfill with two small children. I reluctantly gave up my standard of cleanliness. Ideals fell from godhood with a remarkable thud. I joked about wishing I could love being a disastrous housekeeper, similar to a friend who could keep food and art materials spread out on a kitchen counter for days. After a while it was difficult to tell which was food and which was art.

Ambitions and ideals seem to push and pull, exhilarate or depress our emotional feelings. If our goals are beyond our reach, they will devastate future potential, future dreams. Our compulsion to fulfill every expectation is the road to believing we are defective. Have you planted a standard that is beyond striving, beyond achievement, and beyond hope? If so, then you have accepted deadly ambitions and ideals. They sap your creativity, passion, sense of play, life. They destroy respect for your unique self. *Where perfection goes, your spirit dies, piece by piece.*

Although the *voices* and I have high aims and ideals, some children begin life never expecting much of themselves. Years pass with floundering, limited ambition. Their hands reach out, devoid of energy needed to create life. There is no beginning, middle, or end. This tragic stilted spirit represents a different story, a less familiar circumstance for me since the *voices* and I share mutually ambitious legacies. Others write about the spirits who can not reach goals or ideals, certainly not a richer essence, because no creative force has been implanted either by birth or by experience. For these spirits the music never played.

Damage from perceived, failed ambitions is different for all of us. The understanding that none of us escapes a sense of deficit is one strong mutual bond. Today perfectionism is a serious struggle for young women who assume many difficult roles; wife, mother, career, family support, on and on. There is no way to feel whole, adequate, and authentic.

Psychodrama, a therapy technique, portrays in dramatic format the child's emotional conflict with a parent and is similar to a play with scenes repeating again and again. We know our own dialogue with our parents by heart. Many of us never stopped wanting parental acceptance, parental love, even when our parents have died. We seek approval in the outside world where what we seek absolutely cannot exist. Have you gone to extraordinary lengths to build ambitions and ideals to please and gain acceptance from your parents, peers, or mate? Mates become wonderful recipients of the same desire to gain love and approval needed from our parents.

If we squeeze ourselves into another person's mold, we can precipitate a lifelong crisis of anxiety, fear and depression. The struggle to be, to see our self as competent and accepted, to discover our unique goals and ideals, to embrace our soul's worthiness, is a battle worth fighting. My soul would receive a chill that I would remember forever, if I gave up or lost this struggle for my true self.

Self-preservation is linked directly to living who we are, our honest essence. If we put off expression of our authentic spirit for another day, our life is made smaller and smaller. What comes from our heart, not another's, is a powerful resource for maintaining worth and self-love. Can you insist on this authentic spirit, the inner voice? Can you become completely devoted to the discovery of your own gifts, aims, challenges, and ideals, not those of the original powerful family members, or later replacements. Think back, even when you adopted someone else's choice concerning your own ambitions and ideals, you were likely still exposed to critical judgment.

When I reached my early thirties, I finally began to believe that it was not only my family that controlled my destiny. I was creating it myself. I had moved across the country after college, and yet an aura of my family's influence persisted for many years. My desire for total acceptance was reawakened with each family visit. My expectations never matched the events, which always ended in my disappointment. Being the first born, it was my family's directive that I should accomplish everything perfectly; no room for failure. Well, I have lived through many "failed" choices. My parents and I noticed all of these. Not until fifteen years later was I able to grasp the idea that my life belonged to me. Perhaps more importantly, I later appreciated my gifts and accepted the choices *just the way they were, success and failure alike.*

WHAT HELPED ME ACCOMPLISH THIS?

My seeing choices I made as failures added nothing. An idea crossed my path, and it made a profound difference. It was simple — I do the *best* I can at every point in time. If I could do it any better, I would. I began to accept that premise. It removed a huge burden of regret and shame from my shoulders. I knew I had a conscience, and I knew my choices were the ones I needed to make at the time.

In the French movie, *My Father's Glory,* by Marcel Pagnol, an amusing, poignant series of scenes tells us a story, the age-old story of the young son recognizing the failure of his father's omnipotence. He is devastated and humiliated by events in which his father exhibits failure, but he is able to restore a loving confidence in his father despite knowledge that this adult male is less than perfect. The father's return to a state-of-grace in the son's eyes is predicated on a small but powerful moment of pride in accomplishing something valuable for the son. This movie exquisitely described the humanism of relationships that are accepted even though they are far from perfect, a rare presence in our current family life.

Bron has important information about her origins of ambitions, ideals, and parental failure. Although she partially disclaims the inheritance of gifts from her mother because of the emotional abandonment she suffered as a child, Bron applauds other mentors. Some gifts of her mother are forever attached; the mother's gift of music, good taste, being ambitious, and persisting in goals are a few dominant themes in Bron's life. Bron loved her father and dearly respected his kind and generous nature. She perceived him as a more passive person than her mother, and he had enormous capacity to love and honor her. Bron's quiet standards of honesty, ethics, and integrity came from him.

Bron's grandfather, who owned the only department store in their very small mining town, also had a generous spirit and a loving nature. Bron benefitted from both male resources who loved her. Her survival without them would have been very thin, perhaps non-existent. But let Bron tell this part of the story.

BRON: I always saw my father as one of the best kind of men that humankind could offer. You have to understand when I say this, I am really talking about a hyphenated father; it was father-grandfather. I saw that their instincts were good toward humanity and that their scope was large.

I saw them as most generous. It's one of the first things I look for in people. It was an act of generosity, non-judgmental, all inclusiveness, the ability to put their hands out and help anybody. For example, when the store would close on a Saturday night in the winter, my grandfather would keep it open a half-hour late — an hour some winter nights — to bring in some very poor people so that children would not go without coats. Now we're talking about a very tiny town where the margin of profit was very, very small. My grandfather would sell for pennies above what it cost him.

When my father had his first heart attack I remember how much energy was given to him. In the first two-and-a-half days my father received 350 cards from children in the town. There were no places on any of the walls to put the cards. Each child would write because my father always had done something special for them. It was never a question of a merchant with a customer. It didn't have to do with money and purchase. It had to do with the family, the connections of the family, my father really wanting to know how so-and-so was, and did he recover from such-and-such, or the latest mine incident. These connections were his rewards.

As I got older, the sisters of my father used to say to me two things: one, they had never seen my grandfather as gentle with anybody as he was with me. They didn't remember him like that. They remembered him to be a very stern father. I was always curious about that. I always felt a certain kind of jealousy from the aunts because I was so close to my grandfather, and he was so close to me. The aunts loved me, but they were always rather odd to me.

What was it that I evoked from my stern grandfather? I've always thought it was rather historical that my grandfather must have been very worried left with six siblings to raise by himself. His mother died in the Great Flu epidemic. He was very concerned about doing the right thing. He didn't have to be worried about me. I think it was the lift of worry, and he had already prospered.

About my mother, I can be nothing but grateful for her love of music. I knew how to read music before I knew how to read words. One of my father's brothers would play the piano. He would play the piano for her and she would sing. She was a fabulously talented singer. The positive identifications I got from her were a real gift for me. She had a great love of beauty. She had an aesthetic with an enormous ability to combine things that you would never dream of setting next to each other. It always worked. Her gift was totally intuitive. I used to sit with her at auctions. I used to watch her. I have two cut-glass vase pieces that she put together from which she made a lamp. I was with her the day she did that. I said to myself, that is utterly amazing that she would know that those forms would work so extraordinarily together by seeing, feeling and touching.

She was very powerful. I used to hear people speak about her power all the time. She was the oldest in her family. She was the woman that came into my grandfather's house and took charge of three people who were in my father's family. All of the brothers looked up to her.

I remember very distinctly if they had a problem they didn't go to their wives, they came to my mother like the grand wizard.

I had to spend so much effort not being totally overwhelmed by her, being devoured by her. Now you have to remember that is mixed with being told I wasn't wanted. I mean at every opportunity that story was told incessantly wherever we were. It still was, up until the moment she died.

We had working in our house, by the time I was five, a wonderful woman, Katherine, who also was a model of a human being. Impoverished, undereducated, wonderful, kind, she had every quality my mother lacked. We adored each other. She was a haven for me.

My mother would talk or let you know that she thought she was extremely beautiful and talented. By the same token, somehow I got a sniff that it was not the whole truth. She was a narcissist and she was terribly vulnerable.

There was a group of women she measured herself against when she spoke. She always came out on top but there was something that said she really didn't believe this.

What did I get? I was thinking in terms of what I lost. But I think I spent so much of my life either trying not to be her or in warding off the words of not being wanted. I think I lost a lot of strength that I might have had about who I was. Because she presented herself in such a powerful way, I always felt as if I had to take a back seat. If I wanted to do something right or morally correct or something to help somebody, I would have to do it and then disguise it. I hid the things from her that I did well. I didn't want her to feel as if I were trying to steal something from her.

> **The part of the family that was so strong was the taking care of people. I learned as a very early ethic to take care of the rest of the tribe. You never spoke the "I" word. You never spoke about what you wanted, or what you needed.**
>
> **I would hear my mother say she was going home to her parents. She would walk out of the house and would never say anything to us or tell us when she was coming back. I remember standing silently at the window watching her go across the street to the bus in order to get on the train that took her back to her parents. It was a tremendous feeling, I'm not sure, anxiety — about when she would come back. I was probably very conflicted, I probably wanted to be alone with my uncles, brother, and father, but there was great anxiety about when she would return.**
>
> **I wouldn't have been able to use the word abandonment, but I knew the feelings of it every day of my life. She would wake up in the morning, walk downstairs. Almost always she slept past the time I went to school, but if it so happened that she was up, I remember being struck that she wouldn't say "hello," "good day," "good morning." We didn't get kissed good night by my mother. It was a steady stream into my bedroom of grandfather, father, uncles coming and kissing me good night.**

Bron's powerful, dominant, unloving mother was an instrument of terrible pain. When Bron developed severe colitis in her late teens, abandonment and exposure were continual themes in her life. She lived with fear that her vulnerable essence could be exposed. Everyone around recognized her special talents, her competence in music, painting, politics, relationships. Bron was tremendously outspoken about her values, ideals, and standards, and sometimes presented them as *the* truth, not *a* truth.

Others perceived her outspokeness as strength and dominance. Few suspected the mystery of her abandonment as a child. That small child cried out as an adult for love and respect. Although she received both of these from a spouse, family, and friends, later losses deeply touched her heart. It was as though she could not afford to lose any loving friend or family member. Eleven deaths — both parents, extended family and friends — died during the last ten years. The early deficit of her mother's unloving care had created a deep hole. All new wounds to the heart threatened her very existence. These deaths taxed her emotional life.

When I taped Bron's story, some aspects resonated with my own life. We both had mothers who dominated everything, and we had passive but caring fathers. Our mothers were larger than life, shrinking the confidence and self-esteem of their daughters. Both mothers saw themselves as beautiful and talented, but their original family systems produced doubts and major insecurity about who they really were. In very different ways the mothers passed on their insecurities, anxieties, and lack of worth. Accepting their daughters as they were was impossible, thus creating emotional wounds even the loving fathers could not heal. I remember my mother telling me, at age eight, that a distant cousin had asked her how such a beautiful woman could birth such an ugly child. That ugly child was me, not my brother. Understandably, Bron and I struggled to achieve a hearty trust in ourselves.

After years of experimenting with different talents and skills, Bron and I arrived at a more peaceful acceptance of who we are. Bron lived near a large western city with access to many colleges and cultural opportunities. Politics always interested her and she found a niche in the local community, raising funds for children. She discovered painting and she describes it as a passion and a need. Teachers were available at a number of small community colleges. These became a life line to Bron's restoration. Music (Bron plays the piano) is also a strong source of joy in her life. Many small orchestras exist in her immediate environment, and these allow her monthly opportunities to hear concerts. Her husband, who plays an instrument for some community orchestras, shares in this great love of music. Finally, therapy was always important for Bron. She found a wise elder mentor/therapist who journeyed with her now and again over the years.

My life has similar reference points. Art, both painting and sculpture, remain important aspects of my creativity. I also love restoring old houses and redecorating them. Gardening has become a passion for me. I have a need to balance intellectual pursuit, writing, and creative imagination. My two brains (left and right) dance. I, like Bron, have found a mentor/therapist in the last few years. And, I find music a constant source of joy. Finally, Bron and I had difficult parenting experiences, both as children and as adult parents ourselves.

Beyond the parenting we receive, there is a greater complication to achieving our richest ambitions and ideals. Icebergs and humans have much in common. The major portion of each lies hidden beneath the surface: in humans, that means it's in the unconscious domain. As we illuminate these deeper invisible parts, our sense of risk increases. If our persona were simple we would not struggle against exposure and vulnerability. But it's not simple. We are many different, contradictory selves, many "I's", some hidden, some visible.

I understand spirit as the energy of my soul. The words "Spirit" and "Self" evoke in my mind the largest, most complete picture of who I am, my whole being. That essence, if one were asked to describe it, is difficult to express. It is the *mystery of the Self* that surrounds ambitions and ideals, in fact, *all we are and all we can be.* Why do I use the word "mystery?" The unconscious aspect of ourselves creates a mystery concerning behavior, thoughts, and feelings. Caught unaware, like a deer transfixed by a car's headlights, we are startled at the intersection of our self and another. Only the unconscious holds the answer to some feelings, thoughts, and actions.

From my own perspective, the most difficult aspect of our essence is our unconscious psyche. It lives in the darkest recesses, speaking to us in fantasy, intuition, dreams, and visions. Unconscious spirit can create heart-pounding fear and confusion, as well as leading us into major transition and transformation. Each of these, both fear and transformation, live side by side as we walk our path. It is our responsibility to solve as much of the mystery of the unconscious as we can.

Do you believe you are capable of understanding the contradictions of yourself, the mysteries? The gold mine is your unconscious. When you pay attention to fantasy, intuition, dreams, and fleeting awareness, in the largest sense, the mystery of who you are is enlightened; you can discover your soul. The rational ego mind may resist, fight for control. But ego is not the path to transformation or the soul's nourishment. The crucibles of our lives unfold best within the territory of the unconscious. When friends use therapy, tarot, astrology, ritual, meditation, yoga, dream analysis, or other more exotic links to unconscious paths, they are attempting to make known that which is hidden from them. These are only additional guides.

Even as we are fearful, fascinated, and repelled by the mysteries of our unconscious, a glimpse of something beyond propels us toward our deeper spirit. That source to discover comes from within us. The internal/external crisis and failures bring the ego to its knees. Our current ambitions and ideals *appear* to disintegrate, to fragment. We cannot work. We cannot relate. Now our unique spirit, lying in a dense, dark pool of the unconscious, lifts up, and we recognize from deep within a source of richer material . . . the vital, creative, expressive, primary material. This richer source is vague, weak at first, but it is the beginning essence of transformation. It is rarely a lightning bolt. There is first a small awareness, then more powerful intuition, and finally the desire to act on what we know. Transcendence, as fragile as the wings of a new butterfly, moves gently. The mystery of the spirit exposes itself to new light. Love, work, play, and creativity, fragmented and damaged, on another level, *are in transition*! Forms appear, supplying us with freedom and hope. Our intuitive power guides us to these forms, to re-enchantment, to vital transitions of work, love, and play. And beyond this we may be guided to powerful spiritual nourishment. So much of this comes from fear in the beginning. Fear or no fear, some inner source wants to know and pushes on. Change is the universe's answer to stagnation and death.

When my music stopped and I could not rely on finding any joy in doing art consulting, I refused for some time to make any changes. The morass deepened, my spirit felt fragmented. I experienced intense dreams and, later, fantasies as I drove my car from place to place, hanging art. More and more information filtered in as the original wounds of my childhood opened up, revealing themselves to me. Shame, fear, and anxiety played dissonant music as I grasped the notion that I needed to give up major aspects of the life I had once loved but no longer cherished. First there were many small steps of inquiry, then months later, back to college for an advanced degree, taking many classes that set in motion new personal experiences and different forms of creativity. Days became filled with challenges, forcing me into a work schedule I had not experienced for many years. What kept me going was the intuitive guidance provided by my daydreams and occasional visions of the future. Mentors supported my fragile spirit which worked and played with less than full confidence. At this time I understood a piece of the mystery, my inadequacy, a legacy from my mother's childhood. Beyond my awareness my vitality and creativity were giving birth to new actions, a new way of life. The wounds of my childhood were not a death sentence preventing re-enchantment. Understanding my mystery and the new ambitions that were emerging changed forever my sense of being inadequate. For me the mystery, which I understood as a shared legacy with my mother, was dealt an incredible blow with each new act of my competence. I was becoming the therapist that always existed within me. It was a returning to my essence, the heart center. As Dr. Hammerschlag says "the heart center has no self-doubt."

Our spirit is often restored within a few personal, and fundamental truths. There is not *one* truth but *a* truth for each of us. Transformation and restoration of the self is played out in the field of our deepest unconscious as it returns to awareness and forces us to act.

We catch an intuitive glimpse of the light, and then another, and then another. Strangely enough, what once wounded our child now fuels the re-enchantment of our adult self. The nightmare of childhood lingers, the pungent scent always present, a reminder of our deeper, sometimes tragically shadowed soul. Joseph Campbell put it nicely when he said, "Where you stumble, there your treasure is." Think of Amy, Bron, Raphael, and me. Think of all the *voices.* It is not from our strength but from our flawed essence that we claim our personal re-enchantment and ultimately our music. "Man is born broken. He lives by mending."[4]

Notes to Chapter 4

1. Heinz Kohut, *Self Psychology and the Humanities* (New York: W.W. Norton & Co., 1985), p. 86.
2. Heinz Kohut, *The Restoration of the Self (New York: International Universities Press, Inc., 1977),* p.87.
3. Ibid., p. 312.
4. Ibid., p. 87.

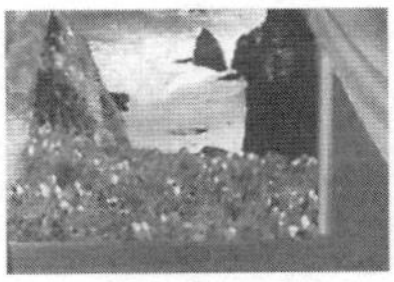

CHAPTER 5

Mirror, Mirror on the Wall

And when she had dressed herself in beautiful clothes, she went to her looking glass and said: "Mirror, mirror on the wall, who is fairest of them all?" The looking glass answered, "O Queen, although you are of beauty rare, the young bride is a thousand times more fair." Then she railed and cursed and was beside herself with disappointment and anger.

ELISSA MELAMED[1]

CERTAIN MOTION PICTURES HAVE A WAY of moving me to a wide open space of character identity. It is as if I step into their shoes or they possess me, like a ghost. For example I feel an unusual connection with several of Federico Fellini's characters, as well as Fellini himself, whose films, he admits, are often biographical. One hero in *8½* is a movie director played by Marcello Mastroanni. His thoughts and intrusions of memories and dreams are projected like misty portraits onto the screen. In a flashback we glimpse his mother and sisters during his childhood hovering around him, attending to his every need. In fact, he is over-stimulated by this attention, often making efforts to ward it off. Though the hero, from childhood to the present time, is emotionally isolated, he is surrounded by people. His mind and physical body are cluttered with the chaos of these relationships. He sees himself reflected back in a hundred of their mirrors. I can experience his internal isolation, which is piercingly and profoundly lonely. In scenes from his later life, I instinctively want him to make some connection — with his wife, a lover, someone! People are everywhere, yet, I know there will be no connection, no empathic relationship and no attachment. In this way he and I are profoundly different.

Fellini's characters frequently lack the very qualities of intimacy the director's real life represents. Perhaps, he came to know these contrasts of isolation and intimate relationships from the dark side of his youth. As I write this I know I am projecting my own identity onto Fellini, imposing myself like a ghost. I can only imagine why he is so fascinated with characters who are lonely, alienated, isolated. His film leaves me with a mystery that I wish to solve in my own life. How did Fellini become the intimate family member if he was isolated in his early life? I ask the same of myself.

Here is a possible explanation, at least for me. During my first eight years I was an only child living in a large city. I spent many hours playing alone or reading books. Some of these books were fairy tales where the female character is rescued from distress by a daring handsome hero. I lived in this fantasy world of rescue. There were opportunities at this time to play with a group of children. Sometimes I played, but more often my mother preferred me to stay home, since it turned dark very early during the long winters. Fantasy games and creative projects with paint, crayons, in fact any art materials available became my way of life. I remember these days and nights as lonely, my father absent much of the time, due to the long commutes to his work, and my mother preoccupied with her own survival.

We moved from the city to a small New England town when I was eight. At our new home I searched for a close friendship, and found one. Through my friend Anne I acquired a second family. I wanted desperately to feel part of a warm, responsive family whose members were together daily. I remember how I felt during my first Christmas with this friend, buying small gifts, decorating a tree, experiencing the warmth and excitement of wrapping presents purchased with my meager allowance. I decorated my first individual tree, placed in a sacred space in my bedroom. My friend Anne was a wise advisor in the celebration of Christmas. Her mother baked enormous numbers of cakes, cookies, and Christmas pies, filling the house with delicious aromas. My new sense of family and friendship would forever after be associated with all the holiday smells.

My baby brother, who arrived just as we moved from the city, became my mother's center of attention, and she divided her time between his care and helping my father with an active local drugstore and old fashioned ice-cream parlor. At times my brother's care became my responsibility, and so as a young girl I soon began to feel isolated from my friends. Later, in high school and college, I reached out for more permanent relationships. To this day I maintain contact with friends I met during those years. Out of the isolation of my childhood I finally developed some carefully chosen friendships.

It was because of this legacy of early isolation and later need for intimacy and connection that I identified so strongly with Fellini and his characters. The director portrayed in *8½* was over-attended and I under-attended, which for opposite reasons created the same experience of isolation in childhood. As an adult, my life has become very different from the movie character because connecting has become a way of life. Some deep core part of myself knew about isolation, a mystery I inherited at my birth. I developed friendships by opening my heart. Now I choose times to be alone so that I might better understand how to live freely and creatively.

We cannot erase the earliest themes of personal identity that come from our parents and care givers. Who are the spirits that mirror your being back to you? Who are your models; with whom do you identify? Imagine a slowly-developing Polaroid picture. Who do you see as your images emerge on the paper? Perhaps you'll believe you see your mother, father, teachers, colleagues, siblings, aunts, uncles, friends. Each image affects you in a different way. Some come and go; some remain there always. Some may betray us, even those in whom we've placed great trust, and as often as not, they do so with complete absence of malice. Some may create safe environments, environments of trust and love though their efforts may not be enough to deflect the pain and damage inflicted by others. Our vulnerability and experiences of betrayal will collude in a dance of self-doubt but our adult awareness of the origins of this dance can help us change the way we view ourselves. In time the image we see can please us, giving us an accurate picture of who we are. *Mirror, mirror on the wall, you are the fairest of them all.*

Even when we have experienced betrayal we may continue to identify with those who least deserve our trust. We may become so spellbound by their actions that we merge our spirit unconsciously with them or others like them. But identifying or merging with another does not necessarily mean being intimate, or forming a healthy and fulfilled relationship. Indeed, we can be isolated and feel very alone at the same time that we are copying or merging with part of another's identity.

A question often asked in therapy is this, "Can I change the identity and influences I've absorbed from my parents?" Each of us has a focal point from which we came, originating in our family and our genes. The tapestry will include old threads, tightly woven, of the conscious and unconscious teachings of our family members and, many guides who follow after. Some of our parents' attributes become powerful influences that give our lives direction. Compelling as it is, this legacy of identification nevertheless changes with each generation, leaving room for evolving a positive identity, even under the most dire conditions. Have you expressed to others how much you would give to change some miserable quality or characteristic in yourself? Chronic anxiety is a good example because it is passed along from generation to generation in so many families, stopping the music in its own peculiar way. How many people do you know who have tried seemingly endless remedies to stop anxiety?

Raphael's story represents an old legacy, repetitive family patterns, as well as his new choices to enrich the family tapestry. As he walks the path of his present life, he is aware of the themes that created his suffering. That is not to say he has separated himself from influences provided by both parents. In fact, he shares some positive and negative characteristics that bind him even now to the early care-givers in his life.

RAPHAEL: We had a close nuclear family on the paternal side. We had family picnics that involved the cousins, the aunts, the uncles, a so-called family circle that met three or four times a year. Dad was the patriarch of the family. I think he became the patriarch because he was the oldest boy that was educated.

On my mother's side, I remember my grandmother as being a very warm and generous person and my grandfather as the character — an interesting, humorous, bright man, who after my grandmother's death, shared a room with me and lived with my parents until he died. There are

certain characteristics that I see very clearly handed down from my maternal grandfather. My maternal grandfather was a collector. He would keep the daily paper for years. He was a conserver. He saved all kinds of things. I used to tease him that he was hunch-backed because he always looked down at the floor and he would pick up all these collections of brass objects, thinking that one day he would pick up something that was gold. He was thrifty. He tried to make sure that he would never lose anything. In those days, you didn't have ballpoint pens, you had ink pens. If somebody would need to borrow a pen, he would loan out the bottom of the pen and keep the cap. He had a wonderful collection of caps.

I can only look at how my parents lived as examples of how they were brought up. From that standpoint, my mother is extremely thrifty in terms of her own family system. There is very little giving, very little exchange of presents. My father struggled as a physician, since he was a physician during the depression. My father did not really make a substantial income until World War II. There was a struggling, but we weren't poor.

My parents were extremely controlling people. The I.O.U. was to obey, to be a student, to learn, to go to college, to be a physician. My sister was to become a nurse.

My father taught me to play chess. He taught me how to model in clay. I perceived him as having very little time, and very little interest in playing children's games. All activities involving my father were work-oriented except chess.

My paternal grandfather was a jeweler. He must have been a perfectionist. There is no question that my father was a perfectionist, and extremely driven in a work ethic.

I owed my parents doing things that were acceptable to them. The vivid example was in the area of sculpture. When I was in college, I did some — what I believe were fabulous — sculptures, very emotional in their impact. They were not accepted by my father. One was cast into bronze, on the condition that I make a change so it is less gory (in his eyes). The other he refused to put into a permanent bronze. After that, I just gave up sculpting.

My entitlement was to be a mirror image of my father. I was entitled to do the research that he wanted done. I suspect very strongly, that I was entitled to be the physician that he was, though he professed other choices. I became this physician.

We have this tapestry, of which my father's color was blue. I took the same tapestry and instead of making it blue, which is what he wanted, I made it aquamarine, a shade of blue. But it's basically the same tapestry, somebody who devoted his life to the work ethic. I did the best I could, but during the time that he was alive, the attempt to be different was always met with a lot of negative criticism.

There was a competition on his part, a way of always giving you the message that no matter what you did, he had already done it before, he had done it better, or there was a better way to do it. There wasn't that feeling of comradery in which, if I came up with an idea to do something, you'd get that warm feeling of somebody putting their arm around you and saying, "That's a great idea. I wish I had thought of that. If you need help, let me know, and I'll see what I can do to help you with it." It was the opposite. "Do you really need to do that?"

I saw my parents as two people very much dedicated to each other, very loving to each other, working very closely. A positive legacy has always been to help the other person grow.

Raphael has been able to create change in a few significant parts of his life. His parents had supported him to mature and develop his skills and resources but they had a strong proscription about what these would be, what profession he would choose, the kind of person he would marry, and his lifestyle. The father mirrored only himself to his son. He wanted Raphael to follow closely the same worldview and choices in a medical career. By contrast Raphael's parenting of his own children is supportive of growth: each child is encouraged to create their authentic essence. He believes his children know who they need and want to be.

RAPHAEL: There is probably one story that I can recall that demonstrates how hard I tried not to do to my children what I perceived my father did to me — this control, this feeling of no acceptance to be me, that I had no boundaries to call my own.

My middle one, Cara, was very athletic and competitive. She got into cross country running, which in high school was three miles for girls. The coach wasn't very good, and the girls weren't in the best of shape, but the team did fairly well anyway.

As always, I tried to be at the races, but this time my parents had the first opportunity to see her run. As the girls got to the finish line, one of her teammates collapsed and had to crawl over the line. Cara finished standing up but she was white as a ghost. Dad called me aside and told

me how wrong it was to let her do this, that she would kill herself running. There was just no way that I could have told her that running, this important part of her life, was something she would have to stop. That would be repeating the family system and I couldn't do it. I encouraged her to keep on running, to get better training, to be herself. I had sleepless nights worrying that I, as a father, had a responsibility to my daughter. I didn't want her hurt, but I needed so badly to let her be her own person, something I felt I had never achieved.

Raphael's adult children followed their authentic desires. On the other hand, Raphael's life has closely mirrored his father's. He went to the same medical school and entered the same medical specialty. He was intensely aware of how confined he felt, being in his father's shadow. Always the ghost of his Dad spoke, do this, do that, don't make that choice. Later in life Raphael was an advisor, never the proscriber of choices for his three children. As each child developed, each assumed more and more responsibility for their own unique life. Raphael gracefully withheld his opinions unless asked. From this story we can see that what is painful in one generation can be repaired in the next. The understanding of our legacy and the determination to transform it must be a strong intention or the changes will fail. Like father, like son is not an absolute.

Raphael's parents were joined in their beliefs about guiding him, as well as having shared expectations. What occurs when each parent is vastly different and each wants something from their children that mirrors their own aims and values? A no-win drama begins. The conflicted child may attempt to please both demands, withdraw from either parent, or completely withdraw or rebel from both caregivers. Any choice produces a dissatisfied parent. What are the most severe outcomes? Parents respond in unsympathetic ways or withdraw completely from their children's lives. Parents can demonstrate concern but it is coated with criticism and harsh judgment. Advise and destroy becomes the theme.

If the child is punished for being or for not-being, for acting in one way or acting in an opposite direction, then the conflict may undermine the development of the authentic self. Children can be continually lost and make choices far removed from their preferences, gifts, and the dictates of their own souls. If a child remains invested in attempting to please conflicted, fighting parents, the adult soul is faced with different degrees of annihilation. Our very souls are deadened, leaving no source of joy and abundance. The music dies.

I create a rich existence when I respond to both masculine and feminine identity themes. I can enlarge my true spirit and add wonderful resources. I sometimes go camping and when I do I always feel like a male pioneer — chopping wood, making fires, cooking on a wood stove. Fixing a household machine creates the feeling of being a competent male do-it-yourselfer. Enriching themes are layered one on top of another — creative, sensitive, assertive, logical, technical.

We know DNA is only part of our identity; learning is equally important in the tangled web of nature and nurture, genes and environment that determine the course of our lives. Adaptation becomes a valuable process for expanding who we are. When generations of parents and surrogates send defective pictures about who we are, adaptation allows the child and adult to search for new nurturing relationships. Identifications with empathic, loving, functional people can be added to the hand you have already been dealt. Raphael, Bron, and I adapted because we wanted to survive.

As adults and even as children, we have opportunities to explore new mentors and guides. We can find different mirrors and we can walk a new road. Raphael found teachers in school who helped him develop his integrity, his authentic self. They saved his life.

Bron, who you met in Chapter Four, speaks about the necessity of accepting new guides. Bron went beyond her mother and the family to vitalize who she is. She created enormous adaptations by choosing different mentors, and of course, they also chose her.

> **BRON: I was in eighth grade. All my teachers were Irish Catholic. They were wonderful to me. In eighth grade there was an award given for the brightest boy and the brightest girl. Maybe not brightest, but the ones that performed the best. I remember having absolutely no idea that I was going to win, because in the sixth grade I knew I had the best grades, and the girl with the best grades was not chosen to recite the Gettysburg Address. A student with poorer grades was picked. I later was told I was not picked because I was Jewish. Well, eighth grade came along and the person with the best grades, me, got the award.**
>
> **I remember the day of those awards. My teachers making a big fuss. One even said, "Do you own any lipstick?" I said, "Oh no, I don't wear lipstick." She said, "Would you ask your mother to let you bring some tonight?" On the program I was playing the piano and singing. I thought, "That's strange. Why does she want me to wear lipstick tonight?" Then I wondered, was I not looking good enough for this program. And then she said, "Is your mother coming tonight?" I said, "I don't know." But I knew**

in my heart that she was probably not going to come. I was singing, I was in a play and she never came. All the other parents came. My mother did not come.

I remember protecting my father in a way by not telling him what I was doing. There would have been a conflict if he wanted to come. So, I was taking care of my father. Sure enough, everybody else's parents were there. They filled the whole high school. I won the prize for having the best grades. No one was there for me. It was a terrible, terrible feeling.

My mother really believed that women shouldn't get good grades. There she was, mourning over the fact that she never had a musical career. I was to be a mother, or a wife, or whatever it was she deemed to see me as. She would represent to me that intellectuals didn't make good wives and mothers. On the other hand, after I won that award, I remember overhearing her say to one of my father's brothers, whom we all disliked, "I want you to know that Bron won the award for being the brightest girl in the class," and there was utter disdain in my uncle's voice for my having done that. I won the award in ninth and tenth grade. She never came. Eighth grade you might understand, that was for practice. She would not come for the ninth or tenth grade: that was real pain.

I was in recitals from the time I was three. That's a part of my life I don't even talk much about. I used to feel like a pet seal, because I was always the youngest, and there was always a tremendous applause. You have to understand that I never felt like me. There was a conflict. I could not stand the gift my mother gave me, which was my singing voice. I remember saying to myself, I'll never know who I am, and who is my mother.

I was chosen at camp to sing the lead in an operatic performance. Those things were looked down on by the rest of the campers. I was always given the leads in the operas. I was about fourteen years old. Then something happened. God knows, I was smart enough to know that the loss was psychological. I had lost all my notes overnight, the five highest notes. I had a very high voice. And they went — they just went. I remember saying to myself, that's not how you lose a voice. You lose a note at a time, or two notes. You don't lose five notes at once. Whatever this is, is major. You must stop singing.

Here's this strength of ego. I think that if I thought of it as my only gift, I might not have given it up. But, I also knew, I had art shows in this little town. This was the nurturing quality of this remarkable coal mining town. The art teacher thought I was something terrific. I used to win everything at school. I was editor of the school newspaper. I was the accompanist for everybody that played an instrument. We used to travel all over the state for contests. I was beginning to get some kind of ego strength. Maybe the first was winning the prize for being the brightest girl.

One of the teachers [a woman I adored] took me in hand. She was my principal in grammar school. She took me aside in seventh grade and said, "Do you know what your grades are?" I said, "Oh somewhere around B's." She said, "Is that good enough for you?" I said, "That's decent." She said, "That's not decent. I have here a record of your IQ. You should be a straight A or A+ student, so I want you to get to work and in the next six weeks I expect all A's." I got all A's, and then I never stopped. It was somebody who cared. That was the importance of a loving teacher. Who knows what I would have done, if I had not

had her. Those teachers have stayed important my entire life. I still see and call three of those teachers.

Bron feared involving her father in her school activities because it created enormous conflict for her since her mother's decision was to not be involved. In the ninth and tenth grade award ceremonies she was left with a soul-wrenching feeling of aloneness. A bright light of hope appeared in the presence of a few teachers who encouraged Bron's true self. Over time her despair was transformed into ego strength and self -worth, as she chose to move away from her mother. But the price of early abandonment shadows Bron's life, taking different painful forms, both emotional and physical. The mother's legacy could have been a mortal blow. Teachers, relatives, friends, a husband, as well as therapy, did much to help Bron develop her wondrous, creative talents in music, art and community politics. At sixty years of age she is a remarkable woman who produces totems of life, large paintings which reflect the pain and pleasure of her years. She connects to friends who support her creativity and intellectual endeavors. Bron most recently went alone to New York City, rented a studio, and painted every day for three months, a stunning act of courage. Creativity sustained her.

What makes the difference between creative survival, like Bron's, or dead ends, like so many people we hear about? I can't establish cause and effect concerning survival and creativity regarding my own life. Yet, my intuition tells me survival and vitality would be impossible now without the spirits who understand and enable me to reclaim my true essence, friends who are themselves vital and creative. I experience circles of hope, one friend connecting to another.

All of us choose unique characteristics and unusual themes from a dazzling range of models. People, places, things, animals, characters from movies, plays and books, mythical figures, and important historical figures can all be the subjects of our identification. We may desperately seek an identity theme hoping to hear our music once again. In therapy, a patient often identifies with a character from a movie or book. This character produces a personal metaphor as the patient walks in the character's shoes, perhaps remembering or acquiring a trait or attribute not previously part of the self. I remember seeing the 1940s movie *Now Voyager,* feeling enormous empathy for Charlotte, the over-controlled, unhappy woman. I further recall my joy when Charlotte became her own person and asserted her essence, separating herself from a domineering mother. For many years that story remained with me as a model, as I learned to assert my authentic self with my mother, and later with other demanding, powerful people. Without these models I am certain I would never have heard the music that has sustained me through so many challenging times.

Although you may choose to identify with all or part of a movie or character in a book, your vision of the character is limited to being an observer or bystander. The fictional character of the stories may be struggling with themes and conflicts similar to your own. In a single moment you may have a flash of awareness, a lifting of blinders, an "aha." Through Charlotte I better appreciated the heavy shoes I walked in as a child . . . troubled, over-controlled, lonely. This movie gave me another sad awareness of my own mysteries.

A film that is frequently mentioned in therapy sessions as a source of identification is *When Harry Met Sally.* We laugh with good humor and tender identification when Sally orders her sandwich. It must contain the right bread, with specific ingredients, and be accompanied by the proper dressing, depending on which ingredients are chosen. Each question Sally asks further determines the exact nature of the sandwich down to the finest detail. That sandwich becomes a metaphor for Sally's life, just as it does for many of us. She strives for complete control, believing this is what will sustain her. What is both poignant and funny about Sally is her desire to make knowledgeable choices, to *control* the outcome of all events in her life. She is clear at first about her identity, but reaches a point when she questions her roles, who she really is. For a brief time, everything seems to be tossed into the air and nothing is certain. What she says she wants, she isn't getting. Without losing her primary sense of self, she must transform expectations of her needs and wants and expectation of others as well.

It is a joyous moment when Sally experiences a new perception of her life, when Harry and Sally accept their fit. We become aware that each has been able to maintain an integrity of who they are, with some variations. Transformation, adaptation, and variations develop over time, — twelve years in the movie. The characters' identifications, their intentions to change specific traits, become acceptable to them after years of collecting experimental data with others and each other. They could never have made those changes without new data and new perceptions.

We never know much about Harry and Sally's families. If we did have that information, we might see how each identified with specified aims and ideals that their parents represented. What we can imagine about Sally's family is a parental theme of being very orderly, scheduled, perfectionistic, fact-oriented and, perhaps, rigid.

At some critical points in my life, I may toss everything into the air and heave some of my identity aside. Clunk. I no longer accept this personality as is — identifications, roles, givens, shoulds, and expectations. I change for the moment who I want to be. I'm tired of being an over-achiever. I change being a housewife and become a dentist. I change seeing my parents weekly. I change being a passive person. But change requires awareness of my inner soul, support from others, and continued experiences to validate the new visions of myself and direction I am taking. People who surround me become important support. I need to choose these associations very carefully. I want to say that again — *I choose these people very carefully.*

Metamorphosis requires time. The process is never immediate. You may flounder, do different things, surprising things. You may begin to collect data about yourself so that the choices you make reflect your true essence. It is an act of courage. Catching a glimpse of your soul, transcending the old stuff is an act of courage. I gave up a driven work schedule and tended a beautiful garden planted over time by Betty — a creative, eighty year old, wonderful being, whose flowers and home I inherited. Her garden helped me create music that had died.

When I am transcending to a richer being, I need time to collect the information. *I need space* to make errors. And most of all, I need to be non-judgmental about my so-called mistakes I have made or will make. If I am to become assertive after spending thirty years of my life being passive, I may need time to explore being assertive, perhaps to even act overbearing for a while. I need permission to be "inappropriate." Over time I can learn how to find out what is authentic and true for me. Experiences are necessary to distinguish what works and what doesn't. Support is essential in strengthening my new notions about who I am becoming. The idea of reclaiming and reorganizing one's life is powerful. Many of us love the romantic image of change but the real drama of living an exceptional transformation is difficult to achieve. We all know profound change is possible. Getting there is what confounds us.

Shana's life for a time was frozen in an identity of limited roles, wife and mother, with little else to sustain her essence. When Shana or others ask, can I make changes, frequently, my answer is an impassioned *yes.* But your whole soul must crave such a transformation, wanting and acting what you need to be, knowing what your authentic self requires, acting your soul's destiny.

For many of us becoming what we wish to be is an arduous road. The paths are unique and the acts remain sometimes mysterious. In my life the paths zig and zag. Finally, I look back on the odd choices I've made and say "of course, that's what needed to happen." C. Hammerschlag, M.D., a neighbor who lives in the desert, writes with beauty about his own quest and identity as well as his journey with others. This is something Carl would talk to me about, if he weren't writing these words, as he did in The Dancing Healers:

> *"I find an enclosed rectangle nestled into the western slope. I will stay for awhile. I leave my pack outside, collect two forked sticks and a cross bar. In the sacred place I make a pipe rack and rest my instruments on it. I light some cedar I brought from Arizona. I pray. Prayer is whenever you allow your tongue and lips to move synchronously with your heart without first processing your feelings through your head.*
>
> *The smoke's fragrance bathes me; it separates this place from the ordinary. It removes the lampshades that keep me from appreciating my own light.*
>
> *I pray about friends, family, ancestors, animals, and the dead grandmother. I pray about my future. In the drizzle, I offer the pipe. My life breath is illuminated in smoke; it seems to make the raindrops stop in midair.*

As I sit I wonder how I got here. By what path did I come to this point in my life, in my work?

I think, on the mountain, that in my work as a psychiatrist I am another guide for people seeking vision. I am a guide who helps people process life's experience and find the message within about who we are, what our purposes are, what our paths are. What I do is just another ritualized vision quest. My patients invest my workplace and my ceremony with power; if they believe in my language, in what I know, then they can receive what I have to say to them.[2]

What mirrors now affect your destiny allowing you to hear the music of your life? What can you say about the reflections of family, friends, guides? Are you a love-shy isolated person, similar to Cary? Did you alter the family tapestry, change the mirror like Raphael? Were you helped by teachers to become your fullest self, like Bron?

Some of us walk side-by-side with compassionate guides who know our soul is shallow now, unable to presently grasp a rich wholeness. In past generations, the 1960's to the 1980's, emphasis was placed on overly-dependent "I's" becoming "we's." When we look more closely at life in the 1990's or the twenty-first century, we may see that the heart is a lonely hunter, the mirror reflecting a ghost.

Notes to Chapter 5

1. Elissa Melamed, Ph.D., *Mirror Mirror* (New York: Linden Press/Simon & Schuster, 1983).
2. Carl A Hammerschlag, M.D., *The Dancing Healers* (San Francisco: Harper & Row, 1988), pp. 168–169.

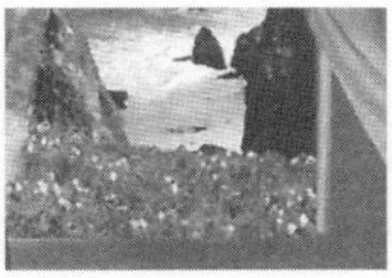

CHAPTER 6

Expectations

My Father says most of the world is asleep, and those who are awake are in a constant state of amazement.

JOE AND THE VOLCANO[1]

When I think about expectations, I especially remember the voice of my mother, wanting me to look neat, clean, and unwrinkled as though I would be captured forever on film. It was a bonus to look pretty but that would not be one of my accomplishments until I was an adolescent. Even then, I had a spotty record, at least in terms of my parent's standards. In my early years — dark, skinny, and pale of face — I reigned as queen of the ugly duckling club, never living up to my mother's dream of having a blue-eyed, blonde, clean, child.

All of us march to a noisy, old parental drum. As children, we may have been messy, but learned that neatness was required. Our parents' edicts to maintain many different traits sit heavily on our shoulders, defying us to be different. Sometimes these proscriptions produce and orchestrate a massive rebellion in us. No longer will we be quiet, careful, passive, verbal, intelligent, attractive, athletic, intellectual, successful, daring, tough, gentle, skilled with tools, on and on, by demand. From our child's perspective, parents represent powerful orders, visible or invisible, to stay in tune with their desires.

At best I find it difficult to know to what extent my parents' damaged legacy is a *cause* of my own pain. In what ways, I wonder, does it contribute to those times when the music stops? I understand some of the obvious settling of fears and anxieties on my accessible soul, but beyond that I am not sure. There are too many variables that make it impractical to predict how I or anyone else will develop.

Amy is a clear voice about negative maternal influences. She decided her mother's abusive emotional scenes would not be part of her own behavior and she consciously chose to curb her emotional responses to everything, to contain her feelings deep within herself. Any outsider would have observed a mother and daughter who were vastly different. It was important to Amy that people see her as a thinking, logical, non-emotional person. Her decision had dire consequences for her physical health, and made her relationships with men difficult. When she channeled her hidden emotional needs into her beautifully expressive art, and when she established intimate caring female relationships, her life reflected her truer essence, more harmony and health. Amy writes about life and art but it is the artwork itself, acclaimed nationally, that sustains her.

When Amy spoke to me, it was clear that the portraits of her mother and father are not black and white but are a wide range of grays. Her adult legacy of ambivalence and rage rises from the depths of these deep, dark grays. It is Amy's description of her mother, a picture of a woman with a light, delightful side, and a very dark, frightening one as well, that underscores Amy's despair during her early years.

AMY: My mother was a warm, open, fun-loving person who was a reacher-outer and a bonder. She had lots of friends and enjoyed her social life. She was very beautiful when she was young but she had a dark side.

I don't think she ever really knew who she was in terms of her life. When my father and mother courted, they always told a story; he took her love letters and corrected them in red pencil and sent them back. There was an unwritten scenario, I believe, that she was less bright.

My mother had a withholding mother, and she adored her father. He was the warm, open intellectual. He died when she was quite young. My mother was the oldest sister. Her youngest sister was very dysfunctional and had a much lower self-concept. My mother essentially as a younger woman was pretty, full of fun, and everybody loved her. I think that later on, in her child-rearing practices, her dark side became more apparent. She was really a tyrant. I guess you would call her the cow that gives the milk and kicks it over. My aunt, when I was four years old, said, "Oh, can you come back and be my little girl?" I said, "No, one mommy to spank me is enough."

When I was growing up, she definitely was a rageaholic. That rage didn't come out to anyone except me. I never saw it directed toward the other children or my father. Yet she loved me. In some ways, I was her favorite. She identified the most with me.

There was always fun and excitement around my mother. Life was exciting. She would take us to the opera. She would take us to plays. She would take us to the symphony. She was a lover of life, a beautiful spirit, but she was never gentle. She wasn't soft and gentle and patient at all. She was always a tyrannical person. I loved her. I loved the part of her that made dolls with me, and that took me to fun places, and had things that smelled good in the kitchen. But there was the other part. I never remember any time in my life that I wasn't terrified of her. The physical abuse burned my self-concept away. It has affected my whole life.

I was never taught how to clean my room, or brush my teeth, or take care of my clothes. They were just dumped in the middle of the room and I was yelled at. I've been teaching it to myself in dribs and drabs, but I never knew how to consistently take care of myself.

Mother wanted me to be a good mother, a good wife, a helpmate. I got the sense that — especially later in life — my mother took a real secret pride in my artistic accomplishments. At the end, I became the person she was always afraid to be. She had tremendous talents that were never fulfilled. She had what I have, and that's called love energy. For my mother, it was very narrowly focused on her family and grandchildren.

My father was very cold . . . he had two sides. On the one hand, he was loyal, very devoted, very much of a family man. He was always there. He would help us with our homework, but he was very blaming and judgmental.

Somehow on an unconscious level I got, "Go for it." Now I don't know if I got those words from my father. He really liked achievement. He wanted his daughter to achieve as much as he wanted his son to achieve. It was my mother, who, when I started achieving, would say, "Don't neglect the family," or, "Are you sure you're being a good wife?" Mother's was always more of a double message. She would never give the other part of the message — that happiness comes from your inner sense of purpose. It was always, "You have to behave a certain way in order to make the men happy." The men always had the power. My brother was the big star of the family. I could never be the star. No matter how many articles I sent home, they would never say, "Oh, we're proud of you." They might tell somebody else they were proud of my career, but they would never tell me. Consequently, I always saw myself as a failure.

My parents would have liked me to be successful, both financially and career wise. They believed in self-sacrifice. In other words, they would never say put your own needs before the needs of the family. They would both say, "Don't be selfish. Think of the family first." I really felt everyone else had to be happy before it was my turn.

I think I got a real message of victim. In order to be happy, or in order to deserve to live, I had to serve other people.

I didn't have a self concept. It was burnt away. I felt I wasn't good enough. I had to earn my right to be on the planet. I had to guess at what was normal.

I had spiritual pessimism since I had been betrayed by everybody. As long as I was a clown, as long as I was pretty and charming and fun, people would love me. If I showed my authentic self and my dark side, nobody would love me. Art became my way of finding my soul.

Along with experiences of physical abuse in Amy's family, she received a double message, that was powerful and damning. The parents, especially her mother, honored and respected achievement but women were expected to satisfy the needs of their children and husbands first. Amy's mother echoed this theme. In the 1950's and 1960's Amy and I were taught that getting married should be our first priority. It never occurred to me that I could go to graduate school and earn an advanced degree. We accepted the idea that becoming a housewife or teacher, or possibly a nurse was the goal of our liberal arts education. Certainly we would not become physicians or attorneys. When Amy says, "I didn't have a worthy self concept," my spirit yells "neither did I!"

Amy's family messages undermined any expression of what was truly authentic for her. She refers to spiritual pessimism, like a parental virus attacking her soul. As an adult, Amy discovered what she needed to expect from herself in order to feel vital and alive. She learned what parts of her spirit to develop, what choices could save her from complete fragmentation and destruction. For her, these expectations became a mission, especially the ideal of "doing good deeds." She has turned her middle years into a mountain of creativity and connection. Amy hears her music.

> **AMY: Although I never fully opened my heart or trusted anybody, I got this message: If you really do good deeds you will earn their love and you will get some back. Maybe you won't get it back from that person, but you'll get it back. I would intuitively figure out what the other person needed, give it to them and then wait for something to come back. It worked because I learned how to be very lovable. I learned how to be very charming. I learned how to fill other people's needs. There was an innocence about me. There was a part of me that never grew up. It worked out in the world, it worked with people.**
>
> **I learned the importance of creativity. My mother valued my creativity, and I learned from an early age that the tool of expanding my creative expression would save my**

life. That was where I was always my authentic self. If it hadn't been for my art, I probably never would have made it.

When I was four years old, I felt that I had a special mission in life. I was really chosen. I had a world mission that kept me alive. I used to pray at night. I used to pray to the sky and the earth. I felt like a lot of abused children, I bonded with the universe, the stars, a lot of things that weren't people. I bonded with people only in a limited way, because I was so terrified of not being good enough, or being rejected.

During much of her early life, Amy felt she was not enough. In truth she had created a large body of artwork which other people considered moving and beautiful. She connected spiritually to many people but she gave herself no credit for these talents because the critical dialogue and abuse of both parents haunted her. At the age of fifty she experienced a serious, debilitating illness, which kept her bedridden for almost two years. Various therapies, Eastern philosophy, diet, alternative medicine, and personally exploring new dimensions of herself, led to her recovery. She spoke, painted, and wrote about her healing process. Today, partly as a result of this illness, Amy has gained respect for her unique spirit, and the tortured dreams and depression she once suffered rarely recur.

As I think about my own life, I can identify with Amy. It is as if our inner lives are dominated by critical committees who sit around and judge us. Even when I realize I am chairman of the board, and have seniority over them, the carping continues. Just allow one doubt about my conduct to surface and the committee informs me that I've just committed a massive error and I fall into a cavernous hole. I expect never to make a mistake. "The critic I abhor is the one (*inside or out*) which is always measuring, comparing, cautioning, and advising prudence and warning against mistakes and quoting authorities and throwing dry, anxious doubts into everyone, by showing them just the way they must go."[2]

Have you fully absorbed the internal critical committee? Has your judgmental nature like Amy's, become so internalized that it seems impossible to fend off its attacks? Many of us constantly *compare* and *measure* our adequacy. Our self-critics sit heavily on our shoulders, disputing our every wish, need, and decision. It draws our attention to every failure and says, "See, this is proof you are not good enough." It exacts retribution, and we are left doubting our integrity and experiencing failure, which fulfills the committee's prophecy and expectation. The enemy is both within and without, internal and external, a combination difficult to fight. The soul reels, primarily from internal forces pressing us to the edge of despair or even bodily harm. Amy's perceived failures took the form of an autoimmune illness.

Can we change this burdensome critic? Only with deep resolve. Questions we must repeatedly ask are, "What priority in my present life requires me to act? What must I do? What must I not do? What action or way of being is compatible with who I am?" When I satisfy my heart center, which has its own vital ambitions and expectations rooted in my authentic self, then I can destroy or at least lessen the impact of the critic.

When the noise of our lives is shut off during those times of quiet contemplation, our intuitive voice, the voice of our heart center and unconscious self speaks. We hear our authentic self in our fantasies, in our dreams, and in our meditation. We hear it in messages gathered daily from all the expressions of our spirit, as well as from our body, which expresses pain whenever we draw away from our authentic inner self.

It is through this process of quieting ourselves that we connect with our own expectations. But can we expect to simply decide one day to change everything and act differently? Chances are that such efforts at sudden change will produce more devastating futility than we felt at the beginning. Rather, we change by focusing attention on one *small* decision at a time, then acting on it. This kind of focus gives us clarity about where we wish to go, based on seeing and trusting our authentic self rather than reacting to the critic. We must limit how far the first step takes us because too large of a step creates failure. I ask myself with each step, "Can I do this?" My inner voice responds, "This much is possible right now." I may feel a sense of being on the right track, and my decision feels joyful.

There were days when I sculpted or wrote when time had no meaning. I felt swept away. At the end of the day, fatigue set in and would create a distance from my work. I would look back on the day's events, tired but extremely happy. I had invested all of myself in the process, even mysteriously, parts of me I did not know existed. When I walk long stretches of the white sand beaches in Oregon, or tend my beautiful Victorian garden, I feel the same engagement with my spirit. It is my real off-key voice I hear gaily singing, *"I can't give you anything but love, baby,"* as my feet touch and walk across the soft sand. Nothing compares to this joy I've come to expect as I live my true essence.

Introspection, that is, looking inward at the real and ideal self, helps us connect to our spirit. As human beings, we cannot live without expecting things from ourself and others. Expectation functions best if our real and ideal self are not dramatically different. When the ideal is too far removed, we are destined to be disappointed and we fall from grace. An ideal I had was to do everything without flaws or mistakes. I expected something perfect all the time. But the real self will commit errors, will misspeak, will decide something with incorrect data. To do this is not only human but necessary. Often our so-called mistakes actually lead to new insight and directions, an idea proposed by Alfred Einstein whose best work was founded on error. When I accept a non-perfect way of being, I bring the ideal self, with its highest standards, closer together with the real self, whose performance is *not flawless.* Only then can I hear my music.

If we hear voices, old and musty, or new and ugly, shouting orders or whispering disappointment about what we should do or we haven't done or could do, we can stand tall and speak with all our inner conviction and truth. Later, as we identify the person we want to be, our voice will become stronger.

I want to talk about the self who is a *misfit*, a *failed stranger*, a *fake*, or a *dark shadow.* We may frequently believe this is who we are. I sit distanced from my true self, watching the pseudo-person, the fake, wondering if the real self will step up. Our fake self is an intrusive thought, unwelcome and defeating and it appears because we do not trust that what we accomplish is completely our own talent. My friend Raphael believed his father orchestrated all his early accomplishments, and so he (Raphael) must be a fake. When he totally left his father's domain and discovered how much his own work was appreciated and accepted, Raphael was able to reclaim a trust in the very real creative person he is.

"I think a sense of individual uniqueness is often hard won. Such a sense is frequently a difficult achievement that is felt as precarious by the individual and that is experienced as a struggle, a struggle against being like everyone else, a struggle to hold together or hold up, or a struggle simply to feel that one has a self."[3] Each of these struggles was a challenge for Raphael, Bron, and Savannah as they walked their chosen paths, even when they were doing what they cherished the most.

Savannah, a special friend of mine over many years, has a legacy that could have annihilated her spirit. Two generations of family ghosts played with her life. Savannah had parents who influenced her expectations adversely, but a strong picture emerges of who Savannah was from the beginning, the strength and vitality awaiting her development. When you read her story it's difficult to imagine building powerful and positive ambitions and ideals after such a lengthy abandonment and chaotic childhood. As her story unfolds, all the clues to the creative, spiritual, and talented evolution of her life become available. Because of the richness of Savannah's life tapestry, I've included more of her story.

SAVANNAH: My mother was a Utah farm girl, one of the black sheep in a fairly large, Mormon family. My parents came from very different cultures. Ellen, being from the farm, which was a very conservative, simple lifestyle. Dad's family had been Southern aristocrats who had marked their heritage back at least to the time of the Civil War. They have always held themselves in very high esteem. They were ensconced in Southern culture that was "Faulknerian," that is, my father was amoral. He was a lover and he was very lovable. He was "in the moment" with how he loved. He was open, not too discerning, nothing that was sustainable. We have letters from before my parents were married and they talked a lot about beer parties. It's real clear to me that their connection was one of acting out, especially for my mother, doing things she was never allowed to do.

They went off and were pioneers for a couple of years. They moved to Nevada where there were houses of prostitution. They didn't have a doctor until my father went

there. Then they moved to Boulder City, which was also a very young town at that time, 1938 or 1939. Most of those people were working on the dam and a few merchants existed. Being the wife of one of the doctors in town was at the high end of the social circle, so that was mother's salvation.

My father was only in my life for about five years. He was in the war when I was born. He came home when I was two in 1945. He divorced my mother in 1950. My father actually lived in the town where we lived for five years after the divorce, but I had no contact with him. Then, when I was twelve he left and I didn't hear from him again for twenty years.

I did feel that in some subtle ways I got a lot of teasing at school. My father married a woman who had children and they were overt in making sure that I knew that they had my dad. Even though there was this patina of being the upper class in a small town, there was also, for the salt-of-the-earth folk that we were very suspect.

The five years that my father was there working as a physician, were good years for my mother. Mostly she was a fanatical housekeeper and a bridge player. She played bridge several times a week. Always for me was coming home from school, the house being filled with smoke, two tables of women who probably had been drinking most of the afternoon. Ellen really enjoyed that. I think it gave her a sense of worth in some odd way. Then, when my father left, he really withheld financial support so my mother ended up working in a drugstore. It was fun for her but very hard and rather demeaning. We didn't have very much money for several years.

There was a war going on between the two of them so there was a lot of very overt anger and hatred coming from my mother about my father. My father, who was this soppy, co-dependent, who wanted everybody to love him, had just created this huge mess. He had an agreement where he would visit us and take us to dinner every Friday night; that lasted two weeks. He would show up at Christmas with tons of packages and that would set off another war. I remember that he used to like to take us to Las Vegas for floor shows. I will never forget playing in my front yard and Dad coming by to pick us up. I was dirty, I had been playing in the mud and my brothers were gone. He was all dressed up and ready to go. My mother had neglected to tell him that we weren't going. It was my job to tell him. It was very hard because I had a very deep love for him.

He was a musician and he really was my model for playing music. I inherited from him a natural ear. He always supported my experimentation with music, having fun with it. My mother wanted to turn that into a structure and lessons.

When this whole thing came down between the two of them, I remember making the choice to take a philosophical attitude; I was seven years old. I remember making a choice to accept who he was and to deal with what was going on with my mother to make it OK in my own head. I don't think I ever grieved. When I was visiting Boulder City this last weekend, I remembered when I was fourteen that we moved from there. This is the first memory that I have of really feeling a loss. When I actually was sitting in my car driving to Las Vegas and seeing that little town of

Boulder disappear. I felt it so powerfully in my gut, it was just the deepest feeling of loss.

Throughout my world with my mother, I identified a loss more with the men in her life than with her. She was insecure, co-dependent, and had very little sense of self in any kind of grounded way. Her sense of self was largely about image, fashion, social status, all those things that were outside of herself. She didn't have much of an inner core. Because of that, she showed up as a quite shrewish person.

One woman, Alice, was my teacher in many ways. She taught me to swim and then she was my English teacher when I was in seventh grade. Alice was an exceptional woman, a pioneer spirit. Everything that came from her was consistent, there were never any double messages. Sometimes these messages were very hard to hear. They gave me a model for consistency and for holism. My family was pretty loose, although we did get more structure when my stepfather joined us at age ten.

I did have a stepfather in my life. Carl was his name. He was a man of German extraction who saved my family in a lot of ways. My brother Steven was five years older than I and was flunking out of high school. My brother Cary was off running wild, getting in trouble with the law as a young adolescent. I don't even know what I was doing. By the time that Carl had been in our family, four years, my brother Cary was on the honor roll and playing sports. Steven changed direction completely. He did so well in college that he was able to attend Harvard for a graduate degree in business. I was a model student but I was always afraid of making any waves. I became too much of a rule follower and gave up a sense of me.

I don't ever remember my Mom being there for me in any substantive way. She gave attention around performing for her. She was a stage door Mom. By the time I was three years old, she had me singing and dancing on every stage in town. I did that for her until I was twelve years old. My life with her was about going to get fluffy little costumes fitted, getting my hair done up, learning how to put lipstick on.

We moved from Boulder City to Las Vegas the summer between seventh and eighth grade which was the worst possible timing for me. I was the ugliest I have ever been. I was used to being the darling of all my teachers and being at the top of my social circle. I moved to Las Vegas and I never recovered. I went into shock around my self-confidence. I never found female friends. I was accepted on a social level, but I never had any kind of an emotional connect.

Carl was very demanding about intellectual pursuits and expertise. I was expected to have very good grades, which I did. I was expected to be adept in the English language, which I am. When Carl came into our life, he had two sons of his own. Those boys stayed with us in the summer. I was good at competing with them. I could hold my own anywhere that skill was needed. I was able to compete in a man's world.

There was a very powerful double standard going on in my home; the boys were all being mentored in the work ethic and getting pay for work. To earn that money, they had regular jobs they did at home. They also worked outside.

My work around the house was every Saturday staying home and cleaning. I was expected to be there to help with meals and dishes, set the table and do some ironing. We ironed all the boys' and Carl's shirts. My mother periodically went to bed for a week with asthma. Then, I did all of it. It wasn't really the work so much, it was my mother's approach to it. The story to me was, women don't get paid for what they do; it's a gift to the household. That has probably been the hardest piece of conditioning for me. I know that I am still dealing with that today, not valuing myself monetarily.

You know that's the conditioning my Mother got. I have a story that really illuminates it. I was visiting up on the farm one year, not long ago. There was this beautiful quilt on the bed that my Aunt had done. I said, "Aunt Ella this is so beautiful, have you ever thought of trying to place some of your quiltwork in a shop?" My Uncle George said, "The women in this house don't work for pay." This woman was a farm woman who had worked from sunrise to sunset her entire life. That was the legacy that my Mom and Aunt Ella passed down. This legacy culminated in my being eighteen years old, a senior in high school, still asking for money every time I wanted to do anything. Mother was in control as to what I could or couldn't do based on whether she was wanting to give it to me. I found out that there were two things that were likely to maximize her saying yes. One was if I had proved that I had been good and the other was if I showed up being needy. That was some very wicked scripting.

What I did in high school was behind the scenes. I took a very powerful leadership role. I was always behind the scenes. But, by the time I graduated from high school, I was voted for three categories in the high school yearbook;

"Most Intelligent," "Done Most for the Class," and "Most Likely to Succeed."

It was me, expressing creatively. It wasn't me trying to be a leader. ("When you got the accolades though, didn't that shift something in you?") I didn't take the awards. I went to the yearbook advisor and I asked her about it. I said, "Is it true that my picture is going to be in there three times?" And she said, yes. I said, "I can't do that." I wanted to choose one of them. I was elected to all kinds of presidencies and I never took any of them.

I just didn't want the responsibility. I think I was carrying so much responsibility in my family, I just couldn't handle it. I didn't have any sense of how to structure. There were some things I knew, the things that Carl had given me. I knew how to keep my keys in my purse. I knew how to find my shoes. I knew how to get good grades and work with my teachers.

I went to school at the University of Utah. That was the beginning of my taking on some thought processes of my own. When I went home that summer, after my first year of college, I started dating Ron, who had been a high school friend. I ended up marrying him the following summer. I was the consummate rule follower, the perfect wife, the perfect mother. I remember shaking in my boots hoping I would be accepted by the PTA.

I learned how to play by ear when I was four years old. When I was about five, my mother took me for lessons to a Ph.D. Music Professor in Las Vegas. I was taught music theory by ear, which was a wonderful gift. I was playing very advanced pieces like "The Fire Dance," I was six years old playing these incredible pieces.

In my teenage years, when I was home alone in the late evenings, I would play. I would play expressively, I would improvise or I would learn pieces from records. For my senior assembly, I decided that I was going to play "Exodus," by Ferronte & Tischer, both pianos. I learned it off the record and I made an amalgamation of their two piano arrangements so that I could do it on one piano. It was the first time that I came out with my music in high school. I was so scared that I couldn't keep my foot on the pedal, and my hands were shaking so badly that I could barely make it through. I had a lot of performance anxiety, especially with the keyboard. Within a few weeks, between that high school senior assembly and when I graduated, I was invited to play with musicians from the school in a little jazz band. I was able to do that. I didn't play piano, I played vibraphone. I was given a vibraphone when I was five years old; I played it in Christmas assemblies, practically my whole life, so I was the Lionel Hampton of the little jazz band and that was good because it prepared me for when I went to college. I actually got a job playing piano in a restaurant during college.

My brother Cary and I went to the same University for two years when I first went away to school and we did a lot of folk music together. During my marriage, once I did get a piano, I learned how to read music. I continued over twelve years to complete my college education and get my bachelor's degree but it was in fine arts. I had an art studio from the time when my kids were very young. Interestingly though, during all of that time, I was still making gifts for the family. I was accepted for a number of really fine exhibitions. I never got grounded in being a professional artist from a standpoint of selling my work.

(You did become a professional musician and write music and record. How did you make that leap?)

It came out of a night dream. In about 1978, I dreamt that I was listening to the radio and one of my songs was on. (I had always written songs since the time I was quite little.) I could see it coming off the tower on the Empire State Building. It was a very exciting dream but I was still focused on my art at that time so it didn't make a lot of sense. I was beginning to play with an art band which was myself, my husband, and four artists. We played at a lot of little alternative venues. I had a good time so music became more present in my life.

It was actually four years later that I had an opportunity to do some recording because Ron had built a recording studio in our home. I had been gone for a year and a half, I had gone back East to New York, a decision that came from the powerful dream about the Empire State Building tower. While I was gone, he built this recording studio and he asked me if I would please come back and give him a reprieve, which I did. I was in the house for three months and while I was there, I thought this is my opportunity, so I recorded an album. Then, I thought well, I'm going to see what I can do with this. I took it to a few local little New Age book stores and they started carrying it. I broadened my horizons and pretty soon I had tapes placed all through California. Then I thought, I might as well get a distributor. By the time I was done, I had twenty-five distributors and I was sending music all over the world and still not expecting to get paid. I could accept the visibility, which was great. I was written up in Billboard magazine and many, many publications all over the world. I have a huge file of the publications. I was played on all of

the New Age stations. At that time, there were about 100 of them all over the country. Very often when I was in Los Angeles, I would hear my music. I could handle the visibility but I never could context it as something that was a business, with monetary value.

Ellen, Savannah's mother, abandoned her when she was very young. Ellen was unable to get beyond herself, her selfish needs, her addictions, her pain. There was also Savannah's father, who was invisible and who disappeared early in her life. Both parents had gifts to give their daughter but the destructive legacies of abandonment, and of not deserving any monetary reward for her work, remained with Savannah until recently. That legacy became an important mystery for her to solve.

Savannah's mother came from a hardy, poor farm environment, simple but determined people, and they passed on an enormous strength to survive. Her father's family was intellectual, bright, talented, musical, sophisticated in their Southern ambience. One aunt, on her father's side, was a brilliant woman who sadly burnt herself out at an early age, ending in her tragic suicide. Destructive themes exist in both parental legacies. We can see the roots of Savannah's strength to survive coming from her mother's family, joined with her drive to excel in many creative ambitions, which came from her father's legacy.

Savannah's relationship with her husband continued for many years, following their divorce. Her transitions from artist, to musician, to originator of a life design seminar program that assists others in finding their authentic creativity and ambition, took place over thirty years. During this time, her husband did not participate in the long journey, although he was a focus for much emotional turmoil. Only recently has Savannah fully recognized the complexity and separation of what is hers and what is her ex-husband's life. When she reclaimed her spirit, with all its pain and joy, her personal expectations were directed by her passionate inner voice. As Savannah sits at the keyboard, she plays her own pieces of music, which are the best metaphor for her present life.

Savannah's family legacy seems on first glance to be nonproductive and damaging. It would be easy to focus on abandonment and despair but then we would miss how she met the challenge and became the creative source of her own accomplishments. Savannah received an enormous gift of musical ability and encouragement from both her father and her stage door mother. She made choices to run with these gifts, no matter what the price. The mother's family legacy of strength to survive gave Savannah the backbone to attempt many new projects. The largest impediment was an expectation of not being rewarded monetarily. In the last five years she asked the questions about financial reward and then demanded her worth directly from clients. She expects to be compensated, and now thirty years later, Savannah is able to enjoy both vitality and financial reward.

If you expect something, you arrange its happening. Perception of events is one of our most important ways to create self-fulfilling prophecies. *If you believe in* some fact or truth about your life, what you *perceive* is likely to follow. You collect data, perceptions, and judgments to fit what you believe is fact. If you believe that people treat you unfairly, you will assure and perceive that people will respond in just that way. It becomes a given that your relationships will reflect this expectation of unfairness. If you believe in a pattern of destructive interactions, such as your abandonment by others close to you, this belief carries enough energy or power to ensure that the expected abandonment will actually occur. Amy did not believe she was lovable, and that belief kept away any semblance of a loving relationship for years.

The following words may be one of the most important clues to why we aren't receiving what we deeply know we want. We act upon our expectations, not on our wishes or wants. There is much power in a wish or want, but we function in terms of what we *expect to happen.*

When I think about the process of therapy, what the therapist changes more than anything else is how the patient perceives the world, what meaning they assign to their life experiences, what they expect to happen. I call this perception positioning of life events. It is what I change as a therapist. One of the stories, told beautifully by Tina, illustrates the process of expectation as it relates to a belief about herself. Tina expected very little for the first twenty-one years of her life; then a traumatic event changed everything. She was able to shift the meaning of her experiences to a positive expectation for her future. I shall call her story *"The Looking Glass."*

TINA: I have always apologized whether I have been wrong or I have been right. And I have done this ever since I can remember. Even if I was right and that person had wronged me, I would go ahead and apologize. It's just like when my father left me, I thought it was my fault. My mother and my father broke up for two years, and my mom had told me that I used to sit up and cry and say, "It's my fault. I wasn't a good girl, that's why daddy's gone."

The bottom line was I couldn't look at myself in the mirror. I didn't want to do anything because, why should I? I wasn't deserving. If someone paid me a compliment, I couldn't take it. It's only been the last three or four years that I have really been able to take compliments.

I was compared with my cousin. "Well, your cousin is doing this. Why can't you be like your cousin?" For a long time, that is all I thought about. Maybe I'm supposed to be like that. I'm supposed to be like her. I'm not doing it right.

My dad never talked very much. He wasn't one that could open up his feelings, or that we could go to and open up our feelings. He was very withdrawn. My mom was the one that was very open. She did all the disciplining as well.

I remember I loved to go stay with my grandma because my grandma wouldn't yell at me, and my grandma wouldn't compare me. I could just be more of me. She would tell me that I was pretty, and she would help me, 'Well, let's try your hair this way, or that way, or let's see what looks good on you."

My other grandma didn't like me. I was afraid of her. I was her only grandchild. When I was about sixteen years old, she had to fly to California for a month, and nobody else in the family could go with her. I had to live in a hospital with her for a month and take care of her. She would yell at me. Then I would call home and I would be crying and upset. I was told that I was being disrespectful. I was to never be disrespectful. I was told to stay.

My mom was good at wanting to fix me. I was always the one that needed to be fixed. My mom thought it was very big for me to go to a counselor. But for her to go to anybody — no way, that was out of the question. Whatever was wrong with her was my fault.

One time in a counseling session(she finally went), I told my mother how I felt about my cousin. And my mother just sat there and said, "I didn't know I did that." And I said, "You did Mom." It was strange because that was the first time I had ever talked to my mother, eye to eye.

It scared me. I think it scared her too. It was always, "I'm the mother and I said so and that's it, bottom line."

Now anytime mom is sick or angry, needs something fixed, or somebody's wronged her, I'm called. Tina will fix it. It makes me feel good doing things for people so that's okay. It gives me a feeling that I'm wanted and I'm needed and people are looking up at me and saying, "Tina can fix it."

It's really kind of weird the way I put the rape in my mind. I was raped and that was, it is, and will always be, a terrible thing in my life. But because that happened to me, it brought me to counseling, which not only helped me get through the ordeal of the rape, but the ordeal of my whole life. Before I was raped, I was nothing. I mean, I didn't think I was anything. Now I know that out of this really, really bad thing, an excellent thing happened. I got to know me. I wouldn't be the person that I am today. I really don't think I would be, because I wouldn't have given myself a chance. I still have a little oldness in me where I get hurt. I carry my feelings on my shoulders. That is me. I have learned that it's all right. If that's who I am, then that's okay.

If something happens, I go to the mirror and I look at myself. I could never look at myself before. That was a big accomplishment. I would look at myself in the mirror and I would say, "You're okay. You're all right. You're okay. You're all right." I couldn't say "You're a beautiful person, and now I can. Sometimes I have to remind myself of it. I'm not perfect but I'm okay for who and what I am today.

Tina believed she was a black sheep or even less, "a nothing," She has transformed many perceptions of herself, especially the good, the bad, and the ugly. Her expectations are more realistic. She expects to be something. She accepts the unique spirit she has always been. For the most part, her personal mirror reflects self-worth because that is what she requires of her life.

"We are so many selves. It"s not just the long-ago child within us who needs tenderness and inclusion, but the person we were last year, wanted to be yesterday, tried to become in one job or in one winter, in one love affair, or in one house where even now, we can close our eyes and smell the rooms."[4] Our heart expects to love and include all that we are on any given day.

Notes to Chapter 6

1. *Joe and the Volcano* — a Miramax movie.
2. Brenda Ueland, *If You Want to Write* (Minnesota: Graywolf Press, 1938–1987), p. 35.
3. Susan Krieger, in *New York Times Book Review,* March 15, 1992, p. 39.
4. Gloria Steinem, *Revolution From Within* (Boston: Little, Brown and Company, 1992), p. 323.

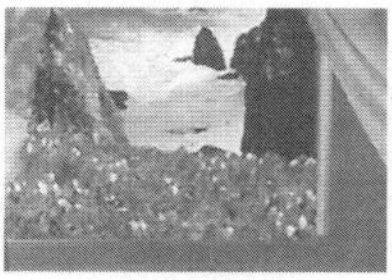

CHAPTER 7

Shame and the Defective One

The Case of the Humongous Conscience

> *The great contradictions which man discovers in himself — freedom and necessity, autonomy and dependence, self and world, relation and isolation, creativity and morality — have their rudimentary traces in even the most primitive forms of life, each precariously balanced between their being and not-being.*
>
> HEINZ LIECHTENSTEIN[1]

ONE OF THE DEEPEST, MOST JAGGED WOUNDS of my life is a feeling of shame when I fail to fulfill all that I've demanded of myself. Hounded by shadows, my energy shrinks as I struggle to fight off my self-inflicted ego and spirit battering. Who was this conscience that told me I'm not enough, that I was a failed parent, and a failed provider? Was it my over-developed conscience that will not accept all that is good? Was it my conscience with no grace, no forgiveness? Was it the conscience of my childhood? Who and what are you now?

When we are ashamed, we do not need other people to express the weight of our shame. We know what event has occurred to create this shame or guilt, and that knowledge is enough to promote pain. In fact, we will very likely have a series of obsessive thoughts, going over again and again what we could have done to avoid or correct the failure.

We experience a loss. What slips away, appearing lost forever, is our *idealized* self. How we failed to live up to a personal ideal generates multiple questions about being adequate. Why is this such a black failure, we ask? We analyze. We question. We wonder. Our perceptions of ourselves seem hounded by a furious chorus of judgmental voices, not just a single critic but a committee of critics. If significant people in our life join this critical self-judging chorus, we are overcome with blame. What about those of us with the *humongous conscience,* an over-developed sense of responsibility for everything, an over-caring experience, a blast of deep, wrenching feelings leaving us battered and naked? The internal demons surround us, knee-deep, and we are judged without mercy.

Savannah knows what it is to be hounded by a chorus of judgmental voices, not the least was her own. She shares a poignant insight about the shame that accompanied leaving her children and husband while creating a musical career in New York City. The good girl she had always been was finally wiped out. It took many years to reconstruct her life, to give up the depth of shame that layered Savannah's soul.

> **SAVANNAH: I was repeating my father's move which was to abandon his family. I knew, I felt that in my bones. When I was doing it, I had a huge grief, I had a huge shame. I took on the burden of the shame around it. I let myself be scripted out as the one responsible. I internally took on a huge guilt and I did it all based on dream imagery. I was making my life choices on the level of the**

> **collective unconscious, not having a clue why I was doing those things. It was like my unconscious was the thing that was leading me. I had no conscious rationale. The other thing that was going on was that I created such a depth of shame in myself by doing that, the part of me that needed to be the good girl was just obliterated in the process. I really didn't heal until I began to get in touch with the original shame that came out of my dysfunctional family. My initial shock was to take on the shame of my family, Ron's family, the neighborhood, every friend I had; I was just completely ostracized and shamed.**

In some very important ways the "good girl" she'd once been was left in the dust. In order for Savannah to find her creative spirit, this good girl who did everything dutifully had to go. The price was very high and yet, the change was essential. When Savannah went to New York, leaving her husband and children, she was answering an inner call to find a career in music. The good girl roles died during that year and two different depths of shame joined together. Savannah finally recognized the original shame of her parents' divorce and the shame that came much later around her own "fallen" family. She passed through multiple experiences, including divorce and career changes, but she arrived slowly, making her peace with grief and shame. Now and then there are experiences that for her create a shudder of remembrance.

There is a way to confront our bloated critical conscience. At an early stage, we internalize parental ideals, values, and restrictions, just as Savannah did. When we violate these standards, we suffer anxiety and guilt urging us to right the wrong. Proscriptions of the conscience carry the weary weight of guilt, as we go through life trying to correct the all-too-often phantom wrongs. However, at the opposite extreme, without any anxiety or conscience, ideals and values are swept away like dry leaves in a heavy wind.

Shame feels different from guilt and it encompasses every inch of our being. Shame is generated when, as a child or adult, we perceive that we've fallen short of our ideal self. Goals and ambitions, as well as ideals, cannot be left unfulfilled without experiencing shame. Failing parental expectation produces the greatest threat and anxiety in children because the child believes the parent will be disgusted and will withdraw their love. That belief is everyone's worst childhood nightmare and too frequently it becomes a reality.

During my own early childhood, probably at age five, I enjoyed chewing gum. My mother kept a large supply of Juicy Fruit™ in a specific place close to the kitchen stove. I was not allowed to help myself. One day I climbed up to get some, thinking she would not know if I nibbled a little from each stick. My mother thought a mouse had eaten the gum and I never revealed the truth, fearing the worst punishment. My mother put a mouse extermination plan into action which we all suffered through for several months. At that time I attempted to save my *wonderful-child ideal* as I would continue to do again and again. For years my judgments about my ideal self were the source of great sadness.

At the core of all shame is the fear of abandonment by those we love. Can you remember this fear? It is the coldest wind blowing on your heart. We may believe we cannot survive without outside love and approval and so, in fear, we comply and submit, hoping that we will be accepted and loved. Our sense of self can become blanketed in doubt and mistrust when outside acceptance is withdrawn. In a heartbeat what appeared to be a well-functioning person becomes a person who is anxious and fragmented. Our very foundations are thoroughly shaken. The lack of loving acceptance can become a mortal blow. Shame creates the greatest dislocation of our soul when our core dissolves.

Early in my life, I experienced some heartbreaking failures — at least that was how I perceived them. I could not tap dance to save my soul, though I dearly wanted to learn. I felt shame and disgust every time I tried, never realizing that at age seven, I did not have the coordination I needed to accomplish my goals. I was sent back to the class time and time again only to experience failure and shame. The adults around me never understood the depth of my feeling, the humiliation in front of my peers, as I stumbled through, missing most of the steps in every sequence. It would be many years before I remembered these experiences without feeling shame.

If you recall Amy's story, her mother wanted a good, sweet, performing child. Amy needed to become invisible whenever she felt any emotion. She was allowed to express only a small range of who she really was, and so she became an adult who could not soothe or give grace to her soul. When parents like Amy's verbalize direct opposition to a child's identity damage occurs because this parent is saying NO to the child's true essence. Amy was humiliated into being alienated from herself. The humongous conscience raged within, leaving deep holes in her soul, blotting out her music.

How does our humongous conscience develop? Let us first imagine the ego and conscience of the shamed person as the ground floor of their core self. It's like a crowded basement, overflowing with multiple items scattered everywhere — proscriptions, shoulds, oughts, judgments, standards, ideals, expectations, demands, codes, ethics, and on and on. If these items are overwhelming, beyond our ability to perform or comply, we experience a punitive, mean, harsh critic. That's the severe humongous conscience showing up, and if our standards are perfectionistic, or we transgress some ideal or value — like never being demanding — we destroy any possibility of a kind conscience. That was my childhood legacy.

If we live with a humongous conscience, what is it telling us? It is stating that we have no right to make mistakes and there is no leeway to think or act in error. We are not entitled to be human and transgress. Shame tells us that our internal standards, ideals, ambitions, and belief systems are faulty and damaged. In fact, our entire self is perceived as damaged and that's the heart of shame. Shame is not projected at a single event: rather, it is welded ever more firmly to our soul with every perceived failure. And when shame has grown in this way, we can no longer imagine a way to address our mistakes, right our wrongs, cure our errors.

Can we change our humongous conscience? Can we eliminate shame? Only by seeing and knowing the experiences of our shame, only by speaking about them and removing self-judgment. We can exorcize this devil, the meanest judgments, the feelings of not being enough, the self-blame, and the self-condemnation only when we are able to understand the feeling of shame and guilt. I say to myself, "This is my huge conscience. I give myself permission to not be perfect, to make mistakes, to be human, to fall short of my ideal, to know that I will fail." What a relief to accept a higher ratio of error!

Therapists and guides can help you form new perceptions that reduce the battering. Beating yourself up is not allowed. You can learn to direct anger against your blaming conscience, not against your spirit. You mentally stomp around. Bit by bit you silence the ugly voices that have become so persistent in your world.

Often we make an assumption that further complicates the process of shame. We assume that everyone around us has their attention riveted on our deficits, watching for us to fail or make a mistake. We expect that no one suspends judgment of our acts and thoughts. We never relinquish being hyper-concerned about other people's perceptions of us. Other critics, in fact, give us another opportunity to be damned, to be battered by shame and guilt. External judgments may simply mirror our own shamed voices, our own projection of failure or fear of failure. The good news is that the external world of judges stays no more interested in our mistakes than our achievements. In a brief time, it is always yesterday's news.

Are there parents who help their children develop a benign, caring conscience? Yes, but they must be loving, empathic parents tuned into their child's true self. Similar guides of encouragement rather than condemnation will be chosen during our lifetime. Raphael's parents, in the following anecdote, were incapable of recognizing the harm they had inflicted.

> RAPHAEL: **One of the problems of my youth was the constant double messages given to me by my parents. On the one hand, I could be anybody I wanted to become, I could accomplish any thing that I tried to do. The power was within me. Then came the big BUT. There were no boundaries. There was constant invasion into my space. My mail was opened and read by my mother. I was told who to date, and who was not acceptable. I was not allowed to play football, to work in areas that my parents felt did not add to my education, so summers were**

> **involved in intellectual activities, not sports, or other things that children did. I did not have a voice. I was an echo! Sculpture, and I made some nice pieces in clay, was to be acceptable to my parents, or it was not worth casting. I wanted to be involved in research. If not suggested by my dad, it was not worthwhile. Years later it became easy to see where this led. I never felt that I had ability, ability to go to college, to medical school, to be an adequate physician, for I was nobody; that is nobody but this echo. I carried that shame and feelings of inadequacy, of being defective, through a good part of my life.**

Like Raphael, many of the *voices* in this book are high achievers who recognized perfectionistic goals that plagued us — goals that in many cases could have killed us. Many speak about a punishing, humongous conscience living within, setting goals and setting us up for failure. Savannah called that punishing conscience her "good girl."

In spite of this self-destructive pattern, the spirit we *must be, and want to be and can be created.* As time passes, adults can develop a conscience that is benign, one that nudges us to act and think within appropriate boundaries — not a conscience bigger than our life, battering our hearts. We can accept ourselves and move ahead even though we have knowledge that we messed up this time. We can say, with full confidence, it is not the end of the world.

My life attachment to high achievement, as well as a truly formidable idealized self, resulted in surrendering my spirit to frequent emotional beatings. Small things stirred the demons: forgetting an appointment, not being available to a friend, speaking to a group and later believing I had forgotten to communicate some information, thinking I may have offended someone with an honest evaluation of data, being left out, sensing angry feelings and deciding I was responsible — on and on. Many events could trigger my anxiety and a loss of my self-esteem. Years into my humongous conscience I came to recognize when and how I fell away from my grace and comfort. I now examine the reality of who I am, what I am realistically able to give. During therapy, I developed a distance from the perfectionistic demon of my ideal self and developed a more merciful assessment of my errors.

Is the ideal self I have to be created by external forces, culture, and family, or from within our own interior coding like DNA? The answer is both. Within the self is a personal coding to respond to the environment in a unique and particular way. My DNA coding, I believe, was originally a perfectionistic expectation to always maintain excellence in all things, and to respond with anxiety if ever there was a lapse. Regarding my environment, I did accept external pressures — social, familial, and cultural — in order to maintain a stable identity. My mother always decided that any problem between another person and me was my fault. Blame was a common word in my family. Any sense of an ideal, blame-free self was, in fact, completely non-existent.

Our identity, who our real self is, remains unfinished as we add more movements and variations to our music. We do recreate our lives again and again. The important message is not the changing identity themes or the repetitive patterns but the acceptance of ourselves, the acceptance of our choices, the recognition that they do not all have to produce successful results. This last point is very important. For many high-achievers, even when we succeed, we experience failure. Shame and the humongous conscience dominate because some small aspect of what we accomplished was not enough for us. We are indeed tough editors of our own life's work. Red pencil scratches everywhere!

There is another dimension to the dynamics of high-achievers. When we succeed we fear that it will be the last time, and we will be left empty and desolate thereafter. So we keep pushing the challenge, demanding even more of ourselves. We constantly create new mountains, telling ourselves, "this is not sufficient, I must push harder and achieve more!" Money is not necessarily what drives us, nor is it what can truly satisfy our needs. What we need is to create something different, something more worthy, something that will maintain our feeling of wanting to be useful. We leave our spirits in constant turmoil, pressing them to perform.

We can turn our adult souls toward a new light, a kinder light. First, here is a poorer choice. We can deny or repress all troubling events, believing that in this way we protect ourselves from the feeling of not being enough. We accept this cover-up, denying the facts, thereby trying to escape the consequences of shame. I believe that this adaptation is very unsuccessful. A secret or truth will ultimately find its way into our awareness. Defenses aimed at isolating the shameful data often fail. At some level we know the truth . . . I cannot forget the incident with my mother's discovered mouse. Information cannot be hidden from the self because some new event will provide data to convince us of the same wrenching inadequacy.

What is a better choice? Where is the light? How do we open our hearing to our music? We can share our humanness, our errors. We can share our mistakes with others who are non-judgmental and thus establish a graceful acceptance of human error. We can use deliberate awareness, to know mistakes are inevitable. We can choose friends and mentors carefully, seeking those who truly support and appreciate the best in us.

I sometimes ask the question: "What will your sentence be for this *crime,* and is it fair and equitable punishment?"

Frequently, a patient will say, "I deserve life in prison or death," to describe what most of us would perceive as minor errors or transgressions. Of course, such statements are totally out of proportion to the humanness of the "shameful" event. I remind them, "You are doing the best you can in a world of difficult choices. Seek support because it is one way of unconditionally loving yourself. Mercy and grace are the light."

In the film, *City Slickers,* the hero asks a difficult question: "After all, what is the meaning of life?" All his defined roles have become stale and he has lost his smile. He feels guilt and shame in not providing what he believes he "should." He once felt like a genuine, honest person but is not certain that this self is still alive. His music has stopped. We see him in a poignant and humorous quest to find his lost true self. He must define who he is at the heart level, without false shoulds, and he must decide what is imperative in his life.

The meaning of life is given to him in a metaphor by an old, worn-out, cowboy. That metaphor is a hand with one finger extended that signifies life is "the one." And what is "the one?" The cowboy tells us it is different for all of us, but it is the path or things that are most important to us, those things we feel passionate about where joy is abundant. In *City Slickers,* our hero returns home valuing his genuine self, which he has discovered in the many adventures out West. He sees himself restored. He recognizes himself as a new person close to his ideal of integrity, kindness, and strength of conviction. His authentic true spirit is doing what it most loves to do.

Each of us develops perceptions of our life and we adjust our glasses so that we can interpret what has occurred. As we look back, it may appear a dry, logical accounting, fixed in concrete notions. In reality our lives are anything but fixed. When the fixed aspects of my life were tossed in the air (I left art consulting, my career, and my marriage) I discovered that nothing exists in concrete. Our investment in work and relationships is always alive, moving, changing. Anything can transform, at any time in our lives. Our interpretations will validate or reject what we choose, just as it did for the hero in *City Slickers.* As he grew closer to his true self he rejected being an insincere advertising executive.

We may have chosen relationships, work, or careers that represented who we needed to be at one time or another in our life. We may experience shame or guilt now for what has malfunctioned. We may even be shocked by the incompatibility of our work and our spirit, shocked by the apparent disparity between our ideals and the reality of our life. Those who divorced partners may be ashamed of this perceived failure. If your life was good and then things began to sour, you experienced a fall from grace. Though difficult, turning points such as this are opportunities to transform what appear to be mistakes, into authentic paths and visions.

Shana tells about her fall from grace. The life she had chosen was enormously demanding, bringing her to complete exhaustion. She had to hear her true voice before her time literally ran out.

SHANA: Certainly the inner voice was telling me continually to rest, to take time out, to do this or that. However, I had a drive to remain acceptable and do what I perceived as safe. But that's a paradox isn't it? Right? I mean, you're not safe if you destroy yourself physically. You destroy your health and you can't keep going.

I started looking around and realizing that because of the hours that I worked, because of the state that I was in when I came home, my children weren't getting any

quality of me. And I wasn't able to enjoy the quality of them either. Everything was too busy. Everything was being pushed and driven. All of those questions and answers started coming up very, very clearly, saying, "Guess what? Change the game again." In my life I had done that many times, very dramatically.

I literally could not make my body move. I couldn't do it. It wasn't a matter of, "I feel emotionally or mentally depressed, so I am just going to sit here." I physically could not move my body without experiencing such excruciating pain, and such exhaustion. I blacked out in the supermarket a couple of times. And it was like, "How much more do you need to see, Shana?" My friend said, "I am aware that the only thing that is going to help you is to have your world brought down to only you."

When I got the information, I made huge changes, and they were very risky. To me, it would have been a greater risk not to take them. There are those that said they were entirely too risky. Even about the point of stopping the marriage, they said, "Oh no. Do whatever you have to do and stay there." But, you see, I have never been able to do that. When the information comes in, I listen and make the change. I will experience fear and all those things and I will still do it. The other ways are certain death.

I went away for a couple of months. I had to stand up and ask for what I needed, including from my former husband. It was such a shift in the cycle to have me call him, ask him to come over to my home because I needed to tell him some things, ask him some things, to sit down and say, "I'm tired, I'm sick, and I need your help." How could he not hear that? What an experience.

Shana left the world she knew, her children, career, family, ex-husband. She lived alone in Hawaii for three months. That took incredible courage — to leave family and friends, to live alone in a strange new environment. If she had remained, a life-threatening respiratory illness would have killed her. As it was, she could barely get on a plane to seek rest in a sunny climate. When she returned, she was no longer seriously ill. When our backs are against the wall, we choose extraordinary paths.

Shana had lived twenty-five years of her adult life trying to do everything that fit others' ideals: to be the perfect wife and mother, to succeed in a demanding career, to fulfill her boss's expectations fourteen hours a day. Guilt motivated her to perform because no accomplishment was enough. Now, after a lengthy vision quest and spiritual renewal, there were enormous transformations in her personal and business life. Shana discovered a new career which enabled her to take care of her health and her three children without compromising either. She did not have to perform or live someone else's program and at best she discovered the joy and abundance of hearing her music.

Many of us struggle to end shame and guilt when we have fallen into the void of not being our fullest self. If we find our game worth playing, if we live our true essence, if we discover those paths that are joyful and alive, we are no longer catapulted into the holes dug deep by our old humongous conscience. After all, what is grace? For me it is knowing in my heart that I create what I need at this place in time, that I accept my unique design and destiny with all its human failings.

As my life lengthens and the shadow of my mortality rests on every leaf and rock, I am called to make a decision. Do I accept the tyrannical rule of a humongous conscience permitting my demons to chase away the music, the beauty and the joy, or do I trust myself, knowing my unique soul invests all that it can and always the best it has to give. "*Freedom and necessity, self and world, creativity and morality — balanced between their being and not-being.*"[2]

Notes to Chapter 7

1. Heinz Liechtenstein, *The Dilemma of Human Identity* (New York: J. Aronson, 1977), p. 4.
2. Ibid, p. 4.

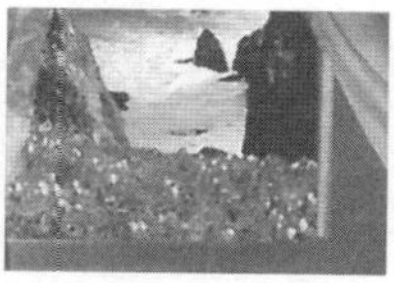

CHAPTER 8

The Game Worth Playing

The Game encompasses the player after the completion of meditation as the surface of a sphere encompasses its center, and leaves him with the feeling that he has extracted from the universe of accident and confusion a totally symmetrical and harmonious cosmos, and absorbed it into himself.

HERMANN HESSE[1]

WE ARE BORN WITH FRAGILE EGOS as well as personal mysteries. A very powerful and elusive vulnerability is created by these mysteries, which may appear as stark as bare bones, or clear and full like a ripe peach. I struggle to understand myself, who this person was, who this person is and yet some certainty about her continues to elude me. I know my survival is deeply affected by my early mysteries, especially those of abandonment and rejection. In fact, my survival often feels clearly like a miracle.

"With some patients, I have the sense of hands raised above the water for the last time just before sinking under; and I cannot dive in and pull them out.... The patient may struggle with his whole will and mind, but yet not make it to the other shore — and succumbs to the crippling conditions of his illness."[2] At times swimming to the other side has seemed impossible. Yet, this is the miracle of those who can swim to the far shore — those spirits born with fragile egos, those voices who courageously speak about their lives after the destruction of birth and childhood, and even beyond the damage of painful adult experiences. I am thinking about Raphael, surviving his overdirected, lonely childhood; Amy transcending the abuse of her mother and sister; Bron's mother repeating she doesn't want a child; Savannah overcoming the abandonment of her mother and her father, and finally myself, disturbed and emotionally unattended enough at age four to attempt a runaway from home, an effort that was halfhearted but frighteningly real.

You may have friends whose early lives are prototypes of tragedy, whose experiences created terrible deficits. In spite of this, they go on, sometimes with passionate initiative and with creative work to produce lives you can hardly imagine.

How and why we survive is as varied as the personal stories of our lives. Resources, mentors, skills, talents, little or large, are utilized by us, always leading us to different forms of creativity and imagination.

Watching kites fly on the Oregon coast one day gave me this thought. The kite flounders at times, doesn't seem to know it can fly, flops on the ground trying to rise up. Suddenly, as though consciousness is involved, it catches the right angle and soars away. Knowing I can develop a creative destiny with the resources at my disposal is greatly empowering. Like the kite, I can flop and flounder and I can also lift and soar.

All the *voices* we've explored so far were able to do that. Emily learned from experience how to build personal goals and meaning within a family of strong, independent, opinionated people. Over the years she has flown many different kites. During transitions, she has journeyed into creative discovery, sometimes pushing her outer limits way beyond what she dreamed was possible. Could she have done it differently? I don't think so. When her music stops, and it has many times, she finds a way to hear it again. Her essence is both creativity and connection. Here is an earlier part of Emily's story, describing her game worth playing.

> **EMILY: I thought when I got married that I would be happy. So I got married and I walked around the house for a week, thinking, "This is happiness?" I kept waiting to get happy and I thought, "This is not happiness. I hate this. This is boring." So, I immediately went to work and started teaching. None of the wives in the company worked, but I went to work. I taught high school. I taught in the 60's and early 70's and that was an enormous help because I really never had a normal childhood, teenage life because I spent my life on the tennis court. I was in my early twenties, and the students were sixteen, seventeen years old. There wasn't much of an age difference. I taught speech and drama, in which I had a master's degree.**
>
> **I was going to graduate school, and was teaching high school. It was exciting because I was doing something creative. I had two lives. I had this wonderful life with all of these teenagers and it was at the time of Haight/Ashbury drugs and free love, communication, and flower children, I loved it. I was fabulous at teaching. It was exciting. It was communication, it was involvement with teenagers, it was involvement with creative thinking. They didn't have their parents so I was their best friend, parent, mentor, that was the beginning of finding my own self. I would go home in the evening to my other life — husband, marriage, stability, love.**

Then we moved to another state. I didn't have anything to do the first week. My children were six and four years old. We bought a little house. I had never had neighbors before. So I thought, well, if I can teach drug-crazed teenagers, I can teach six-year- olds. I went next door and met the lady and said, "Do you have any children?" And she said, "Yes, we have ten."

I told her, "I think I'll teach art." Then I went down the street and this one little Swedish woman had six-year-old twins, so I started teaching art classes the first week after we moved in. I didn't know what to teach. I sent away for three boxes of fabric dye. We had this little basement downstairs and I bought a hot plate. I poured the liquid dye onto these fabrics. I didn't think I could do any art because I can't draw. So I started pouring and teaching. My life changed. Within three months I was in New York selling fabric to big fashion designers. I found something that I could do. I started at the absolute top level of fabric design. I was lucky because the first couple of pieces that I did were absolutely magnificent. I had never even seen tie-dye. But, I knew my pieces were good.

After that I did thousands of yards that weren't very good. But this is important. You think, "I want to be a photographer" and you take three rolls of film and they are horrible so you think, "I have no talent." But it doesn't mean that you do or you don't. It means that those films weren't good.

I am a born teacher. I like to communicate. I love to teach. I probably love to teach because I have that charisma, but I don't know if charisma is the word. I have ingrained from my father, not my mother, that you have to

be interesting. You have to have something to offer. I was taught to go for it.

As an artist I feel that one never knows if one is doing something really well or just missing. It's very difficult to know if you should put on the next color or stop. It's very, very difficult. I thought, "I can't deny this opportunity. I don't want to be just about there, and miss."

Emily's married life brought her to a world where she needed to discovery different games worth playing. Emily was a designer and a fabric originator. Today she is a multimedia artist. She also is president of her own business, unrelated to art in any form. She continues to lecture on subjects that are her passion, particularly Native American Hopi culture. There is no one way that her creativity unfolded. In the early years she refused to be swept away by boredom. What developed as a creative effort in the basement of her first house has continued to evolve into a rich tapestry of life. Emily says she is not always successful in business or art, but she continuously challenges herself to attempt new interests. Her home is filled with wonders of color, form, and beauty. Emily speaks about *adding more, experimenting, risking,* so that you aren't "just about there and miss."

Small steps, even tentative ones, allow us to explore new spaces. If you say, "I can't find a path," permit yourself to experiment, to collect data, taking *small* steps in one direction or another. This is similar to Emily and her adventure with creating beautiful fabrics. She added, she subtracted, she risked in order to achieve the best possible design. Emily collected data with little fear of failing because she believed some of these attempts would provide an interesting journey even when they lacked success. Emily trusted herself enough to fail.

Alexi Tolstoy's life as a successful writer immediately fills us with images of a major game worth playing, evidenced in classic works such as *Anna Karenina*. But, was it always like that for Tolstoy? He, too, had his time of floundering, his time of despair; his dark periods of the soul when the music stopped.

> *In middle age Tolstoy felt himself suddenly assailed by the futility of life and the meaninglessness of the world. He was in excellent health at the time; he could work vigorously in the fields alongside the peasants and then concentrate for hours at his writing desk; he had already won great fame as an author; he was rich; and he had a wife and children who catered to him. Yet with all this, the feeling of meaninglessness struck him with such power that it was almost like the physical sensation of being thrust into a dark sack. Still, with that extraordinary energy and directness that was characteristic of his genius, he flung himself headfirst at this mysterious impasse, reading and pondering all that philosophers and religious teachers had to say about life and its meaning — but always coming out again at the bottom of that closed sack.*
>
> *In the midst of this personal anguish, Tolstoy pauses at one point, turns his gaze from himself to mankind at large, and observes that there are millions of simple folk, like the peasants he knew, who endure hardships, raise families, and pass the torch of life on to their descendants. These people show no signs of faltering in the continuous struggle for the life of the species. They have experienced Tolstoy's question, but have found a response to it through "instinct". . . . Their answer, as Tolstoy puts it, comes through "life itself." And by this response, they are able to stand open to the larger life of mankind, to the past of ancestors and the future of descen-*

dants. They are free to recognize and respond to the most elemental truths of life.[3]

Tolstoy perfectly illustrates the dilemma of living what others judge to be a perfect life while experiencing a descent into hell. When he recognized the simple path of a peasants' life, which was an instinct to remain open to birth, death, love, work, play, he was overwhelmed by this acceptance and response to life. The revelation deeply affected him, dissolving his anguished impasse. Yet, Tolstoy, for all his genius and complex temperament, could not begin to live so simple a life as his peasants. What he could do is capture some elemental truth about his own life as he wanted and needed it to be.

Emily described the disturbing feeling of a "loss-of-self" as being the off season in her life. What she described was a fragile self, unable for a time to participate effectively in the games of her life. I was reminded of a pre-Christmas stay with my children in a lovely old 1930's resort in Santa Barbara. I was alone, a single parent wanting to bring some fun into my children's life. No one was there. The cabins and rooms empty, cabin lights out everywhere, the dining room an embarrassment of people waiting on two tables, the ghostly, lonely quality of being in the right place at the wrong time as I walked the gravel path between darkened cabins. The loss-of-self, like that walk, creates the loneliest, deepest vulnerability and pain. The worthy games seem distanced and unattainable, but this off season is often a prelude to change.

I reclaim my soul with sequences of work, play, love, creativity, sometimes one alone, sometimes all of them at once. Interruptions and endings are part of the story. Why I choose to invest in one game more than another or to stop everything is found somewhere in the mystery of my soul. I am called from within and I answer that call. Perhaps I am alone, walking on a mossy, tree-lined road in Santa Barbara, and my voice begins a quiet song, an affirmation that the lost self, off-season, will find a new path, one small step at a time. I can hear my music once again.

Cassi is Emily's daughter and Kay's granddaughter. She not only adds another dimension to their stories but, at age twenty-five, she represents wisdom and evolution in her own life. I wish I had known Cassi when I was walking my lonely road in Santa Barbara, a single mother of twins trying to find the way. Cassi has a fundamental belief that is a foundation for all her games worth playing — freedom to choose those things that provide personal happiness. Here is her remarkably wise twenty-five-year-old-voice.

> **CASSI: I think my mother has done everything opposite for us of how her parents raised her. We never had to pick up a tennis racket. She said, "Well what school do you want to go to?" She encouraged me to go through all of my phases. I'd come home with black nails and my hair sticking straight up and she'd say, "Great, go ahead, you look cute." I don't think she got to do that as a teenager because she had to play tennis every day. So, when we were growing up we were, "Ok." But she watched us. She was very protective. She had a few set things that she watched like curfew and weight. When we grew up she encouraged us to do everything — join the school plays, do it all — because she didn't get that.**
>
> **My mother carries a negative memory of her father. She won't touch a tennis racket. I think what my mom didn't get from my grandfather is that he never complimented them. He wasn't affectionate. So my mom compliments**

me all the time, like "I love you. You're so cute." That's the kind of relationship she didn't have. She craved it.

I feel my mother has been very strong. I also feel sorry for her and my aunts and uncles. They have all been damaged, wounded by their tennis experience. Her father would take five kids in one car to school and he would not talk to her or acknowledge her because she quit playing tennis.

All her life she has been there for us. When we came home from school, she was there. Every time we went out she was there. You don't think about it at the time but now I think, "God, that was really special."

What I have gotten from her is her ability to express herself, to say, "I love you, take care," I carry that on to my friends. I think my mom's purpose was her children, her husband. We were first. Then it was her parents. And then I think it was her art.

(Cassi, What gives you your purpose?) My mom. My dad, my brother and then my friends. But somebody asked me one time, "What means most to you? What makes you keep going? What makes you tick?" And I said, "Well, every morning I wake up and I have no idea where I am. I'm a sound sleeper. I have to go to my memory every morning — who do I know, where am I, who is my family?" So the first thing I think of is my mom.

(What have you come to expect from relationships?) Stability, because my family has always been pretty solid — understanding, listening to people, and being considerate. I would look for someone who is generous — because my mom is very generous and has a sense of adventure. My dad was very much an adventurer.

There is respect in my family. I don't think everyone understands each other but they respect each other. There's a common ground, a common bond. This is your family, this is your life. Take it for what it's worth. You may not agree but you have to at least try to meet it halfway, respect a person. I think that idea probably came from my grandmother Kay. She did what she could. She kept the family together. They stuck together and it made them close, to be able to handle any outside events.

What I got from my mother was to do the best I can and be the best I can . . . if it's good for you, if you're happy and you're good at it, then continue. I could choose anything I wanted. The goal was to do it well and to be happy with it. I think I could probably deal with most anything. If you try and you give anything an honest effort and understand it, then you can do anything.

The most important thing I would want to be is a pretty stable, solid person. I think I am. I have a sensitive side. I think — also important — realistic and logical. Common sense is part of being a solid person. You can be smart as a book and not have common sense and it doesn't get you anywhere.

My parents gave me enough freedom, even my father — I don't think it was easy on him to give me freedom. One summer I went to Germany when I was eighteen and then one summer I lived in New York. I've done a lot of that. I think it's important because now I get in a job situation, any situation, and I can talk to anyone about anything.

If I fail . . . I look forward to it, because I have been extremely lucky. If I fail when I move out of town, it's

great. That's one more thing I have to overcome and deal with when I'm young and single.

I expect people to succeed and take it to the top. I cannot understand people when they get in certain positions or fade in their life. I always think there's more. It's important to go after it and get taught everything at least once because it makes you more balanced. It evens you out. If you go for the bigger picture, all the little things are going to even out.

Cassi inherits the legacy of her mother, Emily, and grandmother, Kay. She trusts herself by accepting everything that comes her way, meeting it, and dealing with it. She also has an attitude of respect for other people's positions, no matter how different from hers. Emily's message is to be what you want to be. Cassi looks forward to life and she is enthusiastic and eager to try many games worth playing. Her touchstone is her family and relationships and she is tied to her invincible cord of strength, which is the foundation of all her choices. She expects to succeed, to be happy, and that is a rare self-fulfilling prophecy.

"We are continuously transforming ourselves within a community, out of the past into the future, with and within a complex mind, trying always to gain a little more liberty to be what we are becoming."[4] One of the gifts Cassi received from her mother's and grandmother's legacies was to grasp the freedom to develop her true essence. At age twenty-five many parts of her core personality are still forming and she continually discovers new aspects of work and love that challenge her confidence.

Five years later I revisited Cassi's life and there are a few surprises. She has decided on a career in corporate management, and she has partially climbed the ladder of one company. She has lived on the West Coast, but she has decided to accept a career move that will take her back East away from family and friends. In that sense Cassi's life looks similar to the pattern of five years ago; she is willing to risk. While she has been in love, something she cannot yet identify prevents her from marrying. So far, this is a mystery she has not solved. Meanwhile, Cassi has the freedom to choose an independent lifestyle which makes her happy.

Just like Cassi, many of us try to discover the meaning of love. Is it a game worth playing? The written and visual material about love and intimate relationships, as depicted in the media, can be overwhelming and distorted. They tell us in minute detail how to win a mate, how to fall in love, how to keep love alive. The media sends the message that ambitions and ideals would lapse into total failure without a love relationship. Well, perhaps that's one more illusion of life that we can dismantle.

Somewhere in the experience of the male quest for identity, is a garden where man seeks his intimate love partner. Somewhere in the promise of greater completion, wondrous wholeness, is the same garden where women wear their perfumed flowers to attract their men. Each enters the garden with an absolute belief that he or she will decide who, when, where, and how they will fulfill their love relationship. They will decide what the commitment will be, what it will not be. Each believes they can control these choices. Each believes that their freedom of choice will make love a game worth playing. These illusions about love and completion frequently die within the first three months of a relationship.

Love can be an agent of transformation, providing new identity themes. When we're in love we may often feel transformed, and we discover new aspects of our deepest self, or perhaps just a playful person hidden within us. I remember riding a motorcycle on winding country roads, something that appears now, far too risky an act. At the time, I loved the outdoors, the wind, the sense of adventure, even while I felt terrified. I was in love with the young man who owned this machine and it was love that carried me reluctantly but happily to the experiences.

Unfortunately love, all too frequently, is defined emotionally and without conscious intention, as an opportunity to freeze our identity, to become a permanent, same-self attached to another, and in that frozen mold, our growth is stunted and even silenced, like a tree pushing up through wet concrete. Why do I write this? When you choose a partner to love, you also may choose an identity that conforms to this relationship, a fit far from your true essence. A commitment is sealed and any further alternatives are forbidden. The commitment is to be this person, to accept these defined roles, to project a specific personality/identity. For example, I may choose to follow my mate's decisions about fun, what to eat, what kind of car to buy, how to interact with others, where to live, when to visit family. It is not acceptable to later break the bargain I have made or to change who I became in order to live this partnership. In this static, rigid way, love and creative identity will die. When a love relationship remains alive and worthy it includes change, flexibility and different levels of being. It is far from the old model of living happily ever after, just the "way we were." Only Robert Redford can manage that, or did he?

An odd, sad recent portrayal of the female quest for *love, growth,* and *freedom* is found in the movie *Thelma and Louise.* Both women choose death rather than accepting the constraints of their unacceptable life or changing their loveless life as it exists. They do not have a game worth playing and in fact, did they ever have one? There is a curious, brief vitality they find in their mutually supportive identity as Thelma and Louise plan their escape, their us against the world vision fighting external obstacles. We already know their struggle will end disastrously. The car will plummet over a cliff and all will be silent. Long before the violent end, you want to cry out, "Thelma and Louise, get a life!"

There is a great potential for loving relationships to become vital, creative and comfortable, a game truly worth playing. However, having a receptive nature is key. Nothing will happen if our arms are crossed in defiance, locked tightly to ward off change. If we look at the three phases of George Land and Beth Jarmon's growth model for entrepreneurs,(explored best in *Breakpoint and Beyond*[5]), the model applies to relationships as well as businesses. Using the example of a love relationship, let's follow the three cycles of their business paradigm:

In the *forming* phase (Phase I), there is random curiosity: the couple has a willingness and receptivity to explore all possibilities. During this exploration phase, one or both partners will begin to form patterns that are comfortable and the relationship will proceed beyond fascination into some mutual understanding. Continuity may not exist yet, since they will experimentally choose some things and abandon others at random. Yet, there is excitement, challenge, discovery. Most of us are familiar with this falling in love phase.

In Phase II, a relationship with some rigidity of rules is established and "normal" patterns for this couple develop. These patterns, or norms of behavior, are continuously repeated and the couple starts to focus primarily on stability and each other. In the second part of Phase II, one member may express the desire to include others, to disturb their tightly held unity. One mate may require more independence and, perhaps this lover needs a wider range of experience. If this partner precipitates a rebellion, finding the relationship patterns too confining or too dependent, he or she will create a break to the dependent cycle within Phase II. The relationship is then pushed to the wall, to a "breakpoint" — Phase III. Many different elements in a relationship (the same is true in any business) can create a breakpoint. Internal and external forces produce changes that the couple must acknowledge. After awareness, they need to communicate consistently about needs and desires. There is always some movement, even as patterns are becoming fixed.

Breakpoint, Phase III begins: If one partner insists on continuing without change, or remains locked into old patterns, the love relationship at this point will falter. It may die, a final breakpoint. However, Phase III, if successful, becomes an exciting pull into our future. The relationship can accommodate unique and different attitudes and beliefs. It will tolerate ambiguity and unpredictable experiences if the mates are willing to incorporate the best of Phase I, the forming phase, and Phase II. Phase III, when successful, can include those things that have been left out during the earlier phases. The couple will investigate what they are accomplishing together. They will acknowledge separate "I's", solo activities that each creates as needed, but also provide interdependent functions. The interdependent aspect is important because most of us need another's resources and sharing. In that respect, no one is an island unto themselves. During Phase III, this couple will be capable of determining a new relational road map, predicated on the acceptance of change and transformation. Risk is inevitable in this changing venture but vitality replaces decay as the love entrepreneurship transcends suffocating limits. This essence of freedom is what Thelma and Louise could not construct in their ordinary lives.

A Phase III love "entrepreneurship" accepts the anxiety that is present when you expand into unknown, uncharted territories. If we are to redefine or transform ourselves, and change our relationship, we cannot escape being at risk. We can choose and control the boundaries that will provide some safety and personal meaning. We can limit our risks, but what we cannot limit or expand is our partner's tolerance for risk. That aspect alone can create a relationship breakpoint.

Even when there is harmony between my partner and me, Phase III is still a challenge. Some of the choices we make alone or together are off the beaten path, not the terrain you see from the freeway, more like the interesting heart of a country road. Have you ever pulled off to a side trail and discovered something special you had no idea existed? Phase III can lead to an exciting new road map with many such side trails but it requires partners to be flexible, empathetic, and willing to accept some anxiety that usually accompanies new and different choices. We have many years to accomplish Phase III since we are living much longer lives then ever before in human history.

When I reflect on the many times I made choices to change direction — where to live for several months, new creative projects that required my undivided attention, my energy diverted to previously unknown interests — I better appreciate my partner's ability to adapt and empathize with my dream. I felt at risk when my spouse, like Don Quixote on a white horse, immersed himself in his own quest, inventions, and visions for providing a better world. I lived with vulnerability and some fear just as he did when he partnered my challenging but passionate projects. At times country roads we traveled were deep washboard rides, as well as vistas of satisfying, breathtaking beauty. We played our music!

Love is obviously not the only game worth playing. Work and careers are equally powerful aims in life. For some work and career stand taller than having a love relationship. What can I say about work? Is it a reliable source of the game worth playing?

There are many ways we incorporate work or a dedicated career into our daily lives. When we start defining ourselves in terms of our work alone, sustaining an enriched soul is unlikely. Even if work provides a fit with our temperament, it must be vital, challenging, and inner-directed. But how many careers can stand alone, without any other major ambition such as love and play. For most, this single game would falter. The options available within any career or work system rarely provide advancing roles, those roles that allow exciting vistas. You may want to incorporate your ability, creativity, passion, and skills, along with a second track of career opportunity. Many individuals often describe a gray, blunted and trapped quality to their working world, hardly an environment of creativity and opportunity.

From midlife to old age we may increasingly ask questions about the value and personal meaning of the work we do. We may recognize a tremendous pull to satisfy inner needs as we search for opportunities to bring more joy into our work. Perhaps we want work where there are goals and rewards that go beyond pure economics and power, or work that is not a repetitious product. We may want a career that provides intrinsic self-worth and happiness, bringing a sense of purpose into our lives. As we age (we may live somewhere between 80 and 100 years), the material world often becomes less interesting to us than our inner spirit, our relationships, and our personal values. According to a recent New York Times magazine section devoted to aging, family connections, health, and friendships are increasingly valued as we age. When older people were interviewed about their lives, most recalled memories of significant human relationships, not business deals and "bored" meetings.

Our emphasis on career or work can become so unbalanced that the various other chairs we sit in, may be destroyed. Think of all these chairs as various identities or parts of yourself:

friend, family member, social being, hiker, biker, worker, lover, parent, etc. We may frequently think about what chair is missing, or what chair no longer fits the other choices we have made. When young couples are overwhelmed with work, the lover chair goes out the window.

Now and then I find a person whose daily life is balanced and creative. Carl Jung, a famous Swiss psychiatrist, appeared to be such a person. He referred to forty years of age as the "noon of life". If we think about Jung, he surely began and accomplished his creative, most beloved labor during his middle years. Did the careers of medicine and writing supply his game worth playing? What about the personal themes in his unique life? How did Jung weave the threads of career into a personal life tapestry? What about creativity? Jung tells us about this.

> *My life is what I have done, my scientific work; the one is inseparable from the other. The work is the expression of my inner development; for commitment to the contents of the unconscious forms the man and produces his transformations. My works can be regarded as stations along my life's way.*
>
> *All my writings may be considered tasks imposed from within; their source was a fateful compulsion. What I wrote were things that assailed me from within myself. I permitted the spirit that moved me to speak out. I have never counted upon any strong response, any powerful resonance, to my writings. They represent a compensation for our times, and I have been impelled to say what no one wants to hear. For that reason, and especially at the beginning, I often felt utterly forlorn. I knew that what I said would be unwelcome, for it is difficult for people of our times to accept the counterweight to the conscious world. Today I can say that it is truly astonish-*

ing that I have had as much success as has been accorded me —far more than I ever could have expected. I have the feeling that I have done all that it was possible for me to do. Without a doubt that life work could have been larger, and could have been done better; but more was not within my power.[6]

Jung continues: The stories of the Grail had been of the greatest importance to me ever since I read them, at the age of fifteen, for the first time. I had an inkling that a great secret still lay hidden behind those stories. Therefore it seemed quite natural to me that the dream should conjure up the world of the Knights of the Grail and their quest—for that was, in the deepest sense, my own world, which had scarcely anything to do with Freud's. My whole being was seeking for something still unknown which might confer meaning upon the banality of life.[7]

The stability of Jung's family life and his scientific medical career, provided a foundation which could support fantasy, risk and exploration of the unconscious mind. In Jung's words, he had "a guarantee of a normal existence."[8] This normal existence included a highly supportive and extensive family life. Certainly from an outsider looking in, Jung had a game worth playing. Jung makes clear that one of the greatest satisfactions and aims of his life was *the work* which came to him as a "heat of its fires." But, all of his other life journeys, including family relationships and connection to colleagues, were instruments that contributed to his music.

Jung's relationship with Freud was one of his major personal and professional connections and when that relationship faded Jung was free to explore his own unique realms. Jung had his own mysteries to solve. His passion, the heat of his fire, was the work concerning the unconscious mind and the collective unconscious, which today is recognized as Jung's greatest contribution. Clearly, the enormous volumes of pioneering work, as well as his creative art, emanated from his passion. Jung speaks best about his vision and bliss.

> *Without such a vision I might perhaps have lost my orientation and been compelled to abandon my undertaking. But here the meaning had been made clear. When I parted from Freud, I knew that I was plunging into the unknown. Beyond Freud, after all, I knew nothing; but I had taken the step into darkness. When that happens, and then such a dream comes, one feels it as an act of grace.*
>
> *It has taken me virtually forty-five years to distill within the vessel of my scientific work the things I experienced and wrote down at that time. As a young man my goal had been to accomplish something in my science. But then, I hit upon this stream of lava, and the heat of its fires reshaped my life. That was the primal stuff which compelled me to work upon it, and my works are more or less a successful endeavor to incorporate this incandescent matter into the contemporary picture of the world.*
>
> *The years when I was pursuing my inner images were the most important in my life — in them everything essential was decided. It all began then; the later details are only supplements and clarifications of the material that burst forth from the unconscious, and at first swamped me. It was the prima materia for a lifetime's work."*[9]*

---

*This last paragraph is the heart of Jung, and from my perspective, is the essence of re-enchantment. The passionate, creative work, "prima materia," is the personal richer material. It exists in every fiber of our life, and it is within our souls awaiting discovery.

There were many famous voices I could have chosen as examples here, and so I naturally asked myself, why did I choose Jung? I felt an enormous pull to him after seeing two films about his life, as well as reading several of his books. What resonated with me were several things . . . the images of his art; the mandella paintings; sculpture; Bolingen, a summer retreat he built, filled with his unique creativity; his incredible writing about the unconscious, which seemed a failure at first; the pain he endured during his break with Freud; the psychological models he wrote about, which have become so prevalent, even in daily speech — Introvert, Extravert, Sensing, Intuition, Thinking, Feeling. He invested so much passion in writing such a great volume of work. Not the least of his abilities was a direct, empathetic way he had of relating to his patients, at a time when psychiatrists were remote and distant. Finally, I am deeply moved by Jung's ability to maintain close family relationships, and in his travels, to connect to spirits all over the world including extraordinary experiences in Africa and the Southwestern United States, with people vastly different from him.

As you explore vast elements of work, play and love in your life, ask this question: Are work, play, and love, as Jung wrote, the prima materia, the passionate, creative material of your soul? If you were watching a movie of your life, the energy invested in love relationships and work would probably fade in and out. Maybe you'd notice tremendous differences in what you prioritized during months and years of your life. Could you view a still-frame of yourself creating major changes because love or work denied you a sense of passion and self-worth?

We know by now that our ambitions need to produce specific benefits — our music — a reward for the energy we invest. If they don't, we may desire changes. But a mystery exists. Why do we grasp and hold on when a love relationship or a career are way past their prime? Perhaps our own insecurity prevents us from making changes. Within each of us the fire Jung speaks about flares up and then dies out many times over. Risk creates anxiety, even panic. We back away. Yet, each of us has a passion, a fire, connected to our divine essence. We feel it, we want to experience all of it. But have we allowed fear to halt a determined, creative focus?

We are miracles of expression when we absorb for brief moments in time our harmonious center, our mover, the passion of our game worth playing. If you are stalled or stuck, remove yourself to a quiet place where visions and meditation can soothe you. Some small idea will encompass your spirit. Joy rises within you, where nothing existed before. Looking more closely, you know it is the music of a game worth playing and it will propel you to take a vital small step. "The joy of discovering that joy exists, that it is in us, just exactly as life is, without conditions, and which no condition even the worst, can kill."[10*]

Notes to Chapter 8

1. Hermann Hesse, *The Glass Bead Game, Magister Ludi* (New York: Holt, Rinehart & Winston, 1969), p. 403.
2. Daniel Yankelovich and William Barrett, *Ego and Instinct* (New York: Random House, 1970), p. 454.
3. Ibid., p. 433.
4. Ann Swidler, in *Themes of Work and Love in Adulthood,* eds. Neil Smelser and Erik Erikson (Mass.: Harvard University Press, 1980), p. 237.

---

*J. Lusseyran, blinded at age eight, and incarcerated in a concentration camp during World War II, is able to "see" the world as joyful. He wrote about his experiences and with this writing brings us to an elemental understanding of just how small the gift can be when we find the game worth playing and how little the experiences can be that create joy.

5. George Land and Beth Jarmon, *Breakpoint and Beyond, Meeting the Future Today* (New York: Harper Collins, 1992).
6. C.G. Jung, Memories, *Dreams and Reflections* (New York: Vintage Books, 1961), p. 222.
7. Ibid., p. 165.
8. Ibid., p. 189
9. Ibid., p. 199
10. Lusseyran, Jacques, *Le Monde Commence Aujourd'Lui*

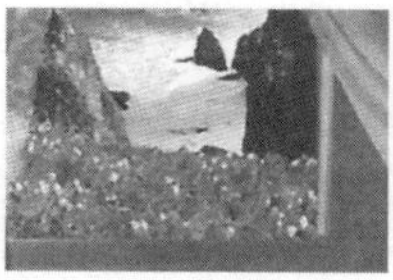

CHAPTER 9

Transcendence—The Dance

We live by attachment, not by reason. That's why love is primary: there is no value without caring, and caring is loving. If, looking about at the world, one finds no one and no thing to love, no bird, no tree, no flower worth caring about, the world is without value; and then, in fatal consequence, one's own life is without value. But if, looking about at the world, one finds someone to love, or perhaps not a person but a dog, or maybe only a plant that wants water and needs sunshine, or maybe not even anything living but a thing, an old house that has sheltered us, that has creaked and moaned in the storms of winter — then one has something to live for, and in consequence one's own life has value only because one cares for others. And one cares without a reason! Without reflection, without the weighing of profit and loss. The caring that justifies everything else is itself without justification. It is a leap.

Attachments grow in the dark, like roots. Silently, invisibly, they extend themselves in heart-soil, anchoring us in the world. To go on living then is not elective; we cannot depart this life, we are held by invincible tendrils

ALLEN WHEELIS[1]

My mortality, my destiny, weighs heavily on me when I have not played in the fields of humor, empathy, my own inner wisdom, and my creativity. And there is also *the dance.* Carl Hammerschlag, M.D., my neighbor, tells a story about this in his book, *The Dancing Healers.*[2] A Pueblo priest and Carl are talking:

> *"Do you know how to dance?"*
>
> *Somehow touched by whimsy at the old man's query, I answered that, sure, I liked to dance; and I shuffled a little at his bedside. Santiago chuckled, got out of bed, and, short of breath, began to show me his dance.*
>
> *"You must be able to dance if you are to heal people," he said.*
>
> *"And will you teach me your steps?" I asked, indulging the aging priest.*
>
> *Santiago nodded. "Yes, I can teach you my steps, but you will have to hear your own music."*[3]

On our worst days we need to know that something exists beyond our pain. We need to know we can heal ourselves and we need to know we can live a richer existence — the passion, the creativity, the joy, all of it! Days or months may pass with little or no "dance." Speaking for myself there is always a possibility that I will respond to the sounds of my inner music, sounds of my vitality off in the distance, forming. This music, I know, will be very tentative at first but it gains strength as I become more fully aware. I attempt a small step and then another and another, and then suddenly, *I am dancing!* As Santiago said, we must be able to dance in order to heal.

Shana understands what Santiago is saying, and she is a spiritual teacher who seeks many forms of achieving inner harmony. When she is part of your life, she shares the rich understanding of mysteries close to her soul. Those who join her seminars, or know her in business, may be surprised by new thoughts and challenging visions she has initiated for them. Let me provide some recent thoughts of hers about what it means to be a transcendent being, or in Shana's words "a divine essence."

> **SHANA: I stood up. The details I won't go into, but I actually stood up as my fully authentic self, a fully empowered woman. My father and I spent time together, we communicated, but he totally shifted off from who I was as an adult woman. He didn't want to hear the details of anything. It lit up too much in him, the work I did all those years as a managing executive . . . in his mind, I was still his little girl, or that very young woman, the secretary. He had no concept of what I did. Every time that we would talk, he'd always say, "How's your work going?" Well great, well fine. "Oh really." He'd ask a couple of questions and all-of-a-sudden he'd say, "Well, I thought you were still working for. . . ."**
>
> **Whenever dad was in a group with other people and he wanted to talk about me, he always retold the stories of me as a little girl. The same stories. They had become what he perceived to be the good times, where life was exactly the way he wanted it. For my birthday, he brought me a lovely card and he literally wrote "I will always remember you as that little girl. . . ." It was sweet, it was beautiful and there it was.**
>
> **When you come from a perspective of self-realization, then it no longer matters what the job is, it matters how you do it. It matters who you bring to it. And that's the reason why I can walk into any circumstance. It doesn't**

matter who the people are. It doesn't matter what kind of work is happening. I can do any of it. The doing part is easy. It's staying present with my essence that makes the difference, makes it rich, makes it whole. If the environment, the relationship, the work, are not conducive to acknowledging that whole, then it's very clear to me, very quickly, that I need to be somewhere else.

When I identify myself as a particular role — a mother only, a daughter only, a child of the parent only, an employee, and any of those roles that have defined lines in my picture of reality — it's like being compressed instead of having the totality of a wonderful presence.

When I talk about essence, I'm talking about the unique expressions, the purest form of who we are. . . . There is so much orientation that I am a little victim that needs to learn, needs to have someone else to give me stamps of approval. Money they pay me. I even have documents that say I've completed courses beautifully. That is all external. Unless I truly step into who I truly am, I'll never feel realized.

The beauty of it — why it's the game worth playing — is because every single time that you allow your attention to go to the expansion not the roles, the essence, stays with you longer.

We are all part of all that is. This is not some flippy, airy-fairy, "new age" deal. What I'm saying is that . . . we are all interconnected. We are all part of the whole. We are not separate. And it's the separation that make us feel isolated, abandoned, and terrified. We are magnificent. And we have come to this planet to do some wonderful things. I can't tell you what all those wonderful things are because they are revealed as you move along. . . .

The people who are grief-, sadness-, or anger-oriented, ask, "Follow my Spirit without hesitation?" I say, "Follow your Spirit." They say, "Why would I try? What difference would it make?" "Well if it would make a difference, how would you like it to make a difference? Are you willing to take another perspective? That's all. Are you willing to entertain another possibility?"

A huge shift has happened. When we look around the planet it's impossible to have been present in the last five years and not have seen that it is, indeed, happening, the shift to wholeness, the shift to our inner essence. Now, that terrifies a lot of people. It has to be experiential, which means get yourself connected with some folks. It has to be the environment that promotes, evokes, and inspires you to investigate and explore who you really are. The accomplishment far surpasses — with so much less effort — what was done before; it equals physical health, emotional, mental, spiritual health. The mastery of expression is fulfilling and expressing more of who we are at the core of self.

"I want to punctuate something," Shana says. We bring our wholeness, our awareness, our true essence to all we do! We are what we express and we can become masters of expression. All of us need people who support our truest self. As Shana says, get connected to those who are not asleep, those inquiring minds who enhance your divine spirit.

Dr. Hammerschlag writes:

The search for truth represents a longing, not a destination. I have come to see clearly that those men and women who survive crises are those who have maintained a special con-

nection to the way. They have walked their own walk with eyes open to the people and the truths around them, without discounting the walks of others. They have developed a special sense of who they are. They have supplemented the knowledge of science with a faith in the mysterious. The lesson they have imparted to me is unquestionably this: if you are going to greet the world as an equal, your feet have to be planted firmly in some unique, prideful recognition of Self. You must learn in a good way that what you are is okay. Then you can know that others are just fine too.[4]

How I experience the world brings me to *a* truth about many things, but not *the* same truth for all of us. If I believe in only one, *the* truth, I diminish respect for the journey of others. But I also diminish myself. When I listen to the truth of others I am expanding, adding to my self-awareness. Spirit is not without mysteries to be solved throughout my lifetime.

When Shana speaks of divine essence and Carl speaks of connection to the way, they are speaking about an inquiring spirit, walking his or her chosen path. I want to include others in my life who are awake to having their own personal mysteries, to those who have opened a door to their heart centers. We solve some of our own mystery in the process. We make connections of the heart. We restore our vital self. And then we become the one who tips the balance in restoring our planet as well. "Healing the planet is an inside job."[5]

If you cannot connect to your truest self, you cannot heal your broken heart, and you cannot hear your music. Adam, a highly successful entrepreneur, was not connected to his heart; he was devoid of feelings. After his marriage fell apart, he described to me the parts of himself that had withered away over the many years he had worked seven days a week. He knew he had invested very little energy in creating a relationship with his wife and child; he had no vital family relationships, no deep friendships, no aim to connect himself to anything but his work. He did not know how he could connect because he felt so much of him had died. And it had. He lived without a heart, existing in a small, suffocating box of his own making.

With the shock of an impending divorce, life stirred within Adam. Emotions he had buried over the years began to bubble to the surface and, at the same time, he became less and less effective in his career. His previous chaotic activity and noise finally ceased. Slowly and painfully he heard a scratchy voice — his inner spirit had something to say. He listened carefully, finally hearing his true voice, a voice he had been missing for thirty-five years. He knew with certainty that it would not be easy to change. The priorities of his world had to be altered forever. Some of the roles he constructed could be transformed. Father, husband, and friend had existed but without a heart. He would rediscover his heart. He chose not to walk back into his old shut-off way of being, even though one foot remained on that ground. It was a shaky position — one foot forward, one foot back. In time both feet would land solidly on his new ground. Adam made a connection and he allowed his heart to lead him to a few loving relationships. Trust came slowly as he opened up, but only in small steps. In therapy, he learned more about himself, and he was able to risk some intimacy with other people. He would slowly discover that hidden deep within his spirit was a capacity for warmth and caring, a capacity to engage his stunted heart in a relationship with his child, and, soon after, other family members. He developed more balance between love and work, and with balance he achieved greater patience and insight.

Like Adam, I am not surprised that love and work, within the tapestry of my life, are primary, interwoven, sometimes unbalanced, and rarely peripheral. How I choose love and work, what balance I maintain within the work/love/play parts of me, and finally what transitions I need to make if I am to enjoy success and abundance, are expressed in the pattern of my life-design. Tremendous introspection and a therapist/guide enabled me to see some truths about this design.

Looking back on the roads of love, play, and work that I have traveled I can see a road map, some routes clearer, large, like freeways, others less distinct, more like country roads that suddenly end. It is a complex map. The paths of work and love always intersect and include creative activity. I frequently find a road to the sea. This is a legacy from my childhood because I have always had a love affair with the ocean — its smells, the sand, sea creatures, and the rolling undaunted waves. I go to the sea for work and peace. It is as though all forms come together and I experience wholeness when I am near the sea.

Work is a major road for me, a freeway I have traveled during most of my life. This is not a strange choice, since work contributes so much to my sense of self-worth. I have never existed without a service-oriented career. It is one essence of my life-design. When one work road ends, another has already taken its place. I suppose you could say that work is my "road most traveled." Emily, Shana, Savannah, and Raphael share a similar life-design. All invest so much of who they are in work as a source of pride and self-esteem.

I like this description of our complex designs: "Life structure is the pattern or design of a person's life, a meshing of self-in-world. Each relationship is like a thread in a tapestry; the meaning of a thread depends on its place in the total design. . . ."[6]

Savannah recognizes the work and relationships that are essential to her true self and those which exist in conflict with her own life design, the ones that corrupt her soul. She has traveled far beyond her earlier tragic experiences and is a master of expression through music, art, computer program design, and teaching. She had a vision of mentoring others to value their own creative self-expression, to become more aware of mind, body, and spiritual development. This is accomplished in a course she devised to explore individual life-designs. Savannah is connected to the way. She writes and performs incredible music; she shares rich relationships, supporting others who walk different paths. Her life now includes spiritual expression, loving connections, and creative work in diverse fields.

> **SAVANNAH: I have always had a great desire and ability to contribute to other people's coming into self. I am self-educated around psychological processes and therapies. What has been magical for me is to learn that my gift is the ability for creative self-expression. That's a big piece that people need and that's something that I live. I have had to discover it and value it. Where I have gotten into the core of my own self-valuing is through creating self-expression in others. There was a lot of living at risk, living on the edge that I had done, since I had left home at eighteen. I have learned how to do that, and how to feel peaceful. It is a gift that I have to share with people right now. The interesting thing is that the structures are breaking down out there in the world. More and more people are in crisis around how to hold what I call creative tension. I know how to do that and I know how to help people do that. So those are two things, the creative self-expression and the holding of creative tension, which are very closely linked.**

> I needed those years of living through them, of experimenting, expressing myself, in order to get to a place where I could understand those as strengths. It's almost like the tragedy in my life, the lack of structure, the anxiety has ended up being my ticket to helping others achieve a life-design. I have something to share with a world that is going to experience much of what I have experienced personally.
>
> I have a clarity of perception that is neither traumatized nor righteous. I can speak from a place of personal wisdom. I don't have to preach.
>
> I'm not in a place of knowing it all. I don't feel like I have to be good. I can be honest. Being good and being honest were always mutually exclusive in my family. I don't have to have a cause, it's not about having a cause. It's about expressing my truth, what is truth for me. I don't feel any need to impose that on anyone.
>
> Also, I built a strong compensatory structure out of spirituality. I always had a strong sense of the spiritual nature of things. Even in my Mormon years, I was very connected to the Christ myth from the love aspect of Christ.

Savannah explored living with risk and feeling anxiety without experiencing total fear. She labeled the fear and anxiety of living on the edge *creative tension.* She uses this tension to express herself in all her chosen work. In this way her anxiety became the fuel for new and exciting dimensions of her life. Like Savannah, many of us can experience creative tension as a means for achieving the visions and dreams we passionately desire. We need to accept anxiety as an integral part of creativity.

Parents are often the beginning, middle, and end force in our life design. The *voices* and I speak about our first exposures to life, which came from mothers and some fathers who provided our ideals and ambitions, as well as a troubled initiation into the world of anxiety. My ambitions to perform and work are directly linked to my parent's work ethic. But none of our experiences are one-sided. Amy's parents created pain *and* they also contributed much to her positive attributes. Amy tells this poignant story about her parents; the design speaks for itself.

> AMY: This is very important. My father got calls from all over the Los Angeles City school system to do people favors and, he always did. He would help them. He would get a microscope for this one, he would get a PC disk for that one, he would give this person a job. He and my mother must have educated thirty young people in their lives. My mother would find the poor, starving and hungry person and she would give them money and educate them. It was like a team approach.
>
> I came from a history, a tradition of mitzvah doing, which is a very high Jewish tradition and I think that quality of reaching out is very, very important when you look at the whole tone of my life. Mitzvah is a good deed, but it's the best kind of a good deed. It's the kind of deed that comes out of empathy, putting yourself in somebody else's shoes and in the happiest way. It's done out of pure love, without wanting anything in return.
>
> Somewhere, there is a larger picture. There's a lot that I got from my parents about loyalty, integrity, devotion, mitzvah doing, caring. There's a very deep, authentic, ethical, and moral value that I think has really helped me. What I didn't get was a belief in a higher power. I had to forge for myself, the God part of it. Both of my parents thought religion was a lot of bunk. There was no such

thing as a higher power, but don't forget when I did the angel's story at the end of my mother's life, she embraced that angel story. The reason she died peacefully was because she embraced my angel.

Amy's legacy includes a moral, ethical, and spiritual structure. There is no way to account for her restoration, her enormous renewal after so fierce a descent into darkness and serious immune illness, unless we recognize her ethical and spiritual beliefs. Her love energy propelled her on a journey to create art. Amy's soul was invested in painting seven enormous canvases over a period of four years. When I stood before her seven huge canvases bathed in light at a University museum, I felt a sense of peace and joy, the rich experience of being part of a wondrous whole. For those moments I merged with the paintings. Many other viewers shared the at-one experience, standing in front of this temple of art, feeling her joy and love as we moved from one painting to the next.

At any age past fifty, our early twilight years begin. Unwelcome thoughts may intrude upon us. Where have I been in my life? What happens now? What vision, if any, exists about my future? The picture we have of our lives is filtered through the lens of our experiences, sometimes clearly focused and sometimes blurred and indistinct. With age our picture becomes tinged, bathed in some unique emotional coloration — anger, joy, bitterness, sadness, regret, happiness, contentment. Just before he died, Jimmy Stewart said, "I had a wonderful life." Frequently, when very old people are interviewed about the important aspects of their lives, an interesting phenomenon surfaces. As we hear or read their stories we may chuckle about the variety of habits to which these oldsters attribute their longevity and even happiness. They have remarkably similar explanations about the causes and the effects of experiences that contributed to their well-being. Many stories include humor. My parents would refer to old jokes and punch lines that broke up their tension or a crisis. "The moral is, if you're warm and happy in a pile of. . . ." and now, my parents in my presence would laugh uncontrollably.

Humor represents a major resource that describes the old person's stable and joyful identity. But humor can also be associated with some terrifying, progressive, debilitating diseases of the elderly. I learned once again from a unique documentary on PBS that dignity, humor, and small happiness are possible even in tragic circumstances. Watching a daughter relate to her aged mother, who had rapidly deteriorating symptoms of Alzheimer's disease, caught my immediate attention. The daughter began to express humor with her mother rather than continually correcting and amending the mother's distorted stories. The daughter called different obsessive periods by name, the Banana period (bananas were found everywhere, even locked in suitcases); the Dentist period, appointments were found on all papers, calendars, even on walls of the apartment. Humor became a way of restoring love and balance to their tender relationship. Humor added dignity to the mother's darkening world of non-comprehension. Many people lose mental and physical abilities during the aging processes and yet these symptoms are rendered less frightening with a more open, lighthearted communication between elderly parents and children. When we create humor, we help provide the music during the last years of our parents' lives and our own as well.

What wisdom do the elders have to offer? They tell us maintaining a creative and active life becomes even more important as time erodes our sharp focus on love, work, and play. Certainly during this last third of my life I can feel some blurring of my mind and body. There is the smallest questioning of my memory, competence, certainty, and of my body's willingness to follow my rigorous directions to perform. I share with others thoughts about the inevitable decline, gaining more acceptance of myself as I learn that none of us can escape the aging process. Of course, I knew that, but emotionally what aging meant was largely a mystery to me until now. I intently seek these oldsters because they are a source of encouragement and they provide some different ways of hearing my music.

Kay at age eighty-five has traveled around the world, stopping in Alaska to visit her daughter and to participate in the famous dog-sled runs. Nothing escapes her curiosity, imagination, and exploration.

When all the *voices* talk about changes in their game worth playing over the past many years, we can understand that the choices they made were not accidental. Bron developed three themes during her sixty years of life: music, politics, and finally art. All of these satisfied different ambitions and ideals. She rejected music as a career two times. First, music mirrored Bron's mother whose desire was to be a singer. Bron had a beautiful voice, but she could not choose any goal connected with this powerful woman who had abandoned her daughter emotionally at every juncture in her life. She turned away from music a second time when her daughter chose to be a musician (she plays the flute professionally). Bron did not want to compete with her daughter. She refused to take away anything that was valuable for her daughter's career and potential happiness.

For a short period politics served a useful purpose in her life. Bron had learned survival skills at an early age. The ability to defend her integrity and to be assertive were essential in political life, just as they were important in Bron's interactions with her mother. Politics also required a sensitive ability to read people, to recognize their agenda and to cooperate with others when it was possible. Bron learned this sensitivity as a child. She ended her political career, a game she, finally, did not feel worth playing. Being less and less invested in politics allowed time to discover other visions related to her true essence. Bron brought her great capabilities and resources to her political career, but her continuing, intuitive awareness and the desire to solve her own mysteries pushed Bron onto a far different path.

> **BRON: I know the one thing that came into play when I thought of going back to music was that my children were very young and showed a tremendous aptitude for music. I didn't want them to compete with me. I didn't want to be in the same field. I was making those terrible comparisons from childhood that I had felt. I literally remember singing and being in concert tours, getting a lot of praise and not knowing if I was singing with my mother's voice or my own. In other words, am I living the life she wanted to live, which was to be a singer? I said no to that. I said no to music, which my daughter chose professionally.**
>
> **The political phase of my life, was for many years, very nurturing. I felt like I was doing exactly what I wanted to be doing. Maybe it was about taking all of the parts of me that I had learned, because in some ways, it's much harder to do politics well than art. If you're doing it well, you're taking more account of yourself, and you have to put into practice, everything you've learned. You're concerned on a moral plane with not concealing essential things or how to reveal some. How to get what you want and need; how to attend to your goals; I've been asked how I knew certain things in political life and I said, "You had to be my mother's daughter." When I was in politics, I could always**

say I wasn't doing it for me, that it wasn't selfish because I was within high, political-sounding moral structures. Starving children . . . you name it on those levels. It didn't have the taste or the smell of being for myself.

I remembered hearing stories of two women that I barely knew in Clatsop County. I remember that I had very strong feelings of dislike for these women who I knew very little about. I got very curious as to why, when their names came up, did I exhibit such strong internal feelings. I didn't know enough about them to know what they had in common. Little by little, I realized that the one thing they had in common was both had left their husbands for periods of time to go paint. And I said to myself, "That is interesting. You really don't hate them, you're jealous of them. That's what you want, more than anything — to paint." And I was forty-seven years old.

So, I began taking art courses outside the house. That forty-minute trip for the first day's class was the longest forty minutes of my life. It was like an eternity. But there was something enormously free in that. When I'm in art, it's joyous. When I'm in it, it's frighteningly joyous because there is such a sense of losing myself. I finally end up saying, "Oh, this process is everything."

Bron found her destiny, sanity, vitality, and joy in painting. Large canvas works are scattered about the house and studio, all filled with Bron's emotional vision. For her to be alive is to paint.

When Tibetan monks visited the San Francisco Zoo, they discovered that a rare tiger had been sick for two weeks; zoo keepers believed he was dying. The monks requested the administrator's permission to chant special pieces for healing. As they chanted over a long period of time, the tiger went up to the area in front of the monks, sat and listened. That same day the tiger began to eat again and now, weeks later, appears to be eating and healthy. Is this true story so different from the healing that occurred when Bron began to paint? Artists are especially sensitive to personal inner needs for harmony, connection, and wholeness. In some different and sometimes unusual ways, our spirits respond like the tiger's spirit to creative efforts as a powerful source of healing.

Creativity gives us the basic clues to vitality or the decay of our soul. Creative people often participate and invest in protecting the environment. They are acutely aware of all that surrounds them, the beauty as well as the corrupt and ugly. Creative spirits have a sense of what is essential in their world, and that is closely akin to the experience of "flow." Flow requires a great attention to detail and a fascination with some creative process. Csikszentmihalyi, author of *Flow,* refers to a rock climber who, as he sets foot on each step up the side of a cliff, notes all the specks of sand in each piece of granite, millions of specks creating one piece of stone. It is a stunning metaphor, it is at once the minute detail and the vast creative beauty of nature — seeing each grain of sand and also responding to the full magnificence of the cliff's beautiful granite face.

When I speak of art and creativity, thoughts of music enter my mind. Music transports me to an emotional world, which I can share with others. It moves me beyond ordinary boundaries to a soothing or exciting experience. I recall a Paul McCartney concert in which he performed many old Beatles' songs. The audience stood and vibrated, resonating mutual emotions: thousands of people feeling, clapping, singing, swaying, dancing. There was a spontaneous response to old memories and the current sound of the music. I believe there is a song for all of us.

As I think once again about the elders, I ask myself, will I grow old with attributes of empathy, wisdom, and humor? Yes, but they take time to develop, and going beyond the need for time, nothing during my life experience has informed me that I can be creative, wise, and humorous without attachments. Surely, loving someone or something is the essence, the heart of all that grows within me. It is my dance. I express undiminished passion and joy during some of the most difficult times, and joy exists then because I have attachments that accompany my soul on all my roads. It was not a surprise for me to learn that symbols of love were found everywhere on the walls of the harshest concentration camps after World War II. In my ordinary life I grasp the smallest, invisible strands of attachment, and they pull me from the depths of crisis to my re-enchanted spirit. It is forever a leap of faith and love. Andrew Solomon, an author writing about the worst struggle of his life, a personal history of depression, restored his sanity with support from loving family and friends, accompanied by much medical treatment for his illness. He wrote this wise thought about his illness, his creativity, and his own music: "The opposite of depression is not happiness but vitality, and my life, as I write this, is vital even when it's sad."[7] Although his creativity died periodically under the siege of dark depression, he now knows his vitality can restore even his most shattered spirit.

When we can explore, adventure, create a series of games worth playing, when we can acknowledge our truest self, when we connect and respect the way of others, and finally, when we discover our richest material, we are dancing. The music is what we alone hear. Joseph Cambell said it well: "If you do follow your bliss you put yourself on a kind of track that has been there all the while, waiting for you, and the life that you ought to be living is the one you are living. When you see that, you begin to meet people who are in the field of your bliss, and they open the doors to you. I say, follow your bliss and don't be afraid, and doors will open where you didn't know they were going to be."[8]

Notes to Chapter 9

1. Allen Wheelis, *The Scheme of Things* (New York: Harcourt-Brace Jovanovich, 1980), pp. 178–179.
2. Carl A. Hammerschlag, M.D., *The Dancing Healers* (San Francisco: Harper & Row, 1988), p. 193.
3. Ibid., p. 10.
4. Ibid., p. 16
5. Mindwalk movie
6. Daniel J. Levinson, in *Themes of Work and Love in Adulthood,* eds. Neil J. Smelser and Erik H. Erikson (Massachusetts: Harvard University Press, 1980), p. 278.
7. *The New Yorker,* Jan 12, 1998, pg 61.
8. Joseph Campbell, *The Power of Myth* (New York: Anchor Books, Doubleday, 1988), p. 150.

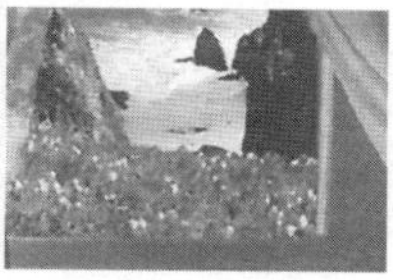

CHAPTER 10

Our Richer Material

A World of Choices

> *At every moment you choose yourself. But do you choose your self? Body and soul contain a thousand possibilities out of which you can build many I's. But in only one of them is there a congruence of the elector and the elected. Only one — which you will never find until you have excluded all those superficial and fleeting possibilities of being and doing with which you toy, out of curiosity or wonder or greed, and which hinder you from casting anchor in the experience of the mystery of life, and the consciousness of the talent entrusted to you. . . .*
>
> DAG HAMMERSKJOLD[1]

BEING ALIVE, INVESTING DEEPLY IN MY LIFE, creates a lightness of being so compelling I wish to remain forever on this journey. Like the astronauts caught up in a space voyage, I feel excited. I know I am on the verge of discovery, some new part of me emerging and growing. There are many times when I experience these periods of passion and vitality, but then suddenly a foreboding enters my thoughts. I awaken in the early morning, feeling some unnamed past pain, mingled with anxiety; my joy is dampened, it's vital edge lost. Half awake, half asleep, I am aware something is changing. Silently, I ask myself a question:

"What happened yesterday that is nudging away vitality and my creative lifeline?" I may go back further in memory so that I can see if a pattern exists. I want to know everything that could produce a shift away from the intense focus on my richer more exuberant thoughts and feelings. There are always some small intrusions, the unremembered dreams hanging over from the night before, or even smaller yet, the dog, the dentist, the yard, the cleaners, the daily tasks that require my attention. I decide permanent bliss is a myth and I will question that myth many times as I watch the changes devouring my creativity. Work, love, play — sometimes separately, sometimes all at once — are inevitably and seriously altered.

From deep within my mind I know anxiety and pain fuel changes and transformation but I ask the question anyway, "Can't I experience transitions without these unwelcome companions?" Answer: "Not very likely." The *voices* and I fit the metaphor of an exotic plant that partially dries up. Our soul survives but some things wither and some things die. Ill winds sweep across our emotional landscape. We have felt them before and we will feel them again. We are on our threshold of change. It dogs us, prods us, pushes us sometimes right up against the wall of despair.

When I shifted my career away from art consulting to private practice as a psychotherapist, my initial responses were anxiety and days of depressing fear. I held onto my art consulting business, working with a few good clients, in the belief that I had to manage both careers. But I was also remembering the joy and vitality of art consulting when it was at its peak. At first I could not risk fully letting go. It seemed beyond my capacity. In the end I did not have the energy required to keep two such vital activities going. I had to adapt and to let go, accepting some losses. My life moved in slow motion as I grappled daily with choices to let go of my old work. Intellectually I knew this was a necessary step but emotionally I resisted this change. I had made changes in my personal life and work before. Where was the knowledge and pattern to make it easier this time around? A truth for my life is that I seem to repeat similar lessons again and again. I am forever walking, sometimes stepping backwards. When I finally make the change, my relief is enormous.

The *voices* and I have spoken about transitions in our lives and we've also referred to incomplete dreams. Kay's box, which included her lost goals, is a beautiful and graphic metaphor, with instructions and insights about adaptation, acceptance, and spiritual restoration. Her life was a struggle, with many adverse conditions, each a form of potential chaos. Raising seven highly independent children was a challenge, especially so because her husband disagreed with her about goals for the oldest children. Her memories are as clear as her startling oceanic blue eyes as she recalls the changing circumstances of the path she walked. Kay has something more to teach me, something that can truly enrich my life. Her *box* provides the space for a transcendent spirit. Within her box are self-expression and freedom, which bring her beyond the borders of the stress and anxiety of her ordinary life.

> **KAY: I taught my children what I thought was important. I wanted to teach them to be independent and to be the best that they were capable of being. And so no matter whatever happened to them, they would be strong enough and ready to face anything. I gave them two gifts, freedom and independence. That was very important to me because I was free. I mean before I was married, I never stayed in one place longer than six weeks. I went to visit my brother, I went here, I went there. I went wherever I wanted to go.**

But once I married, I ended up staying in one place. It was my "box." That's what was in my box. I don't think of it as a sacrifice because you see, in my life I was called upon to do the things that I was capable of doing. Not everybody is called upon to do the things that they are capable of doing. We practically lived as recluses. But you see, I was free within myself. The most important thing to me was that I could create a place to live totally at ease. And I did.

I had all those children and I'm not terribly strong physically but they grew up as individuals. I was juggling all these people with personalities. They're all high-powered, very independent. It was important for me to make it work. I'm sure it could have been done better by somebody else, but it was the best I was capable of doing.

My mother-in-law was very strong but she did not give you the freedom that I gave my children. She was the one in charge and everybody had to come; "you have to come for Christmas — you have to come because I might not be around." Well, she lived to be ninety-six.

I, of course, as a young woman, wanted to do my things because I was used to being independent. Well here I am lumped into this family and you're supposed to be very happy. Well I was happy, but I was not going to be lumped in with the rest of them. I had to be looked upon as an individual, and that I achieved. I demanded that. I got that from everybody. My mother-in-law and I had always gotten along well because I was as strong if not stronger than she was.

You've got to figure out how you can get along with a person. Any place I have ever been, I make this space for the two people. That's actually what happens because I

have to be at ease. That's how I was able to be confined all those years.

I don't ask any more of you than what you are capable of giving. My father wasn't interested in my being the first woman president or the first woman anything. I was basically anything that I wanted to be. I just had to be a responsible person, I had to be strong, and I had to be able to do anything that came into my life. (The box.)

My mother didn't have materialistic feelings or goals, and neither did my father. I think my father wanted to make money to keep us comfortable. What we turned out to be was the most important thing. I have great respect for myself.

We had this old hunting cabin and we went up there twelve to fifteen years ago to spend Thanksgiving. We all had such a good time, that they said "let's do this every year." And I said, "No, we will do it every three years, every third year." That gives them a chance to be with their other in-laws. It gives them a chance to have their own traditions. If my children want to come to me, they're welcome. If they want to do something else, I'm not mad. You're free. That is the most important thing.

(What meaning is there to your life at this point?) What I learned from my mother-in-law was that she — I think of it as a wonderful thing — she was always there. She went to all the children's graduations. She was interested in whatever they did. She was always present. I am always there.

Kay had daily challenges that could have swept her away, driven by stress and despair. Her health was often frail. She gave birth to a large family of high-spirited children whose personalities were as varied as flowers in a Victorian garden. Her husband's return from the war with an obsessive disorder was traumatic and their relationship remained difficult as he pursued a rigid, domineering parental role with his older children. His way of being was contrary to Kay's sensitivity, her concept of freedom, and self-expression. She found herself continually adapting to her husband's demands, as well as sheltering her children from his compulsive proscriptions concerning tennis. As we know from Emily and Cassi this was not completely successful, but as Kay says, "it was the best I could do."

Since her husband's death, fifteen years ago, Kay remains devoted to her "box." Making life work under any circumstances is the dominant theme of her life. But the second theme, freedom to be yourself, permeates all her decisions. She has succeeded in transmitting that belief to all of her children and grandchildren. What is significant, perhaps, is her continued presence in the birth, life, and death of her large family. Kay is the elder wisewoman sharing everything that fills her box with her ever-increasing family.

Daughter Emily's and granddaughter Cassi's spirits reflect several themes: finding a game worth playing; doing the best you can; adventuring into new worlds with your acceptance of some risk-taking behavior; and most important of all, living who you are. Three generations, three souls whose lives burn with a soft intensity of light, three women who hear their unique music.

There's a major thread woven in Emily's family tapestry that is most important for me — trusting yourself. When I trust myself, I make decisions that reflect my soul's inner direction and that's my best source of integrity and bliss.

Like Kay, I am always wanting to choose something that will bring me closer to serenity. I am yearning to establish work, play, relationships, and love that are so healing and complimentary to my soul that I can transcend more of my stressful everyday life.

On any given day we participate in a multi-dimensional reality: hassles with money, the children, work, our health, the boss, the car, our spouse. There is no complete escape from these realities, not for very long. We play out the necessary joys and miseries and these are the passages of our life from one year to another, moving faster and faster.

My spirit searches beyond limited daily borders to a larger picture. There is centered in this *big picture* a vision of my personal, self-expressive, richer essence. I am established in two worlds, the unremarkable day-to-day givens of my life, and the world where my spirit is striving to attain a deeper level. I reach out to communicate thoughts to another person who will understand my creative striving. I want to share ideas and feelings concerning the passion of my richer self. This spiritual connection transcends the mundane borders of everyday necessities and repetitions. I can no more live with a disconnected soul than I can drive a broken car.

Wherever self-expressive, creative tension exists, the richer essence of my passionate spirit exists. If I am to be a transcendent being, I must experience creativity, passion, the fire, and joy. It is essential, not elective. What we do when we hammer a nail, type a page, paint, sell a product, see a patient, teach a lesson, counsel another, is only a part of who we are. What becomes mandatory is living some moments of the day feeling, thinking, seeing, touching something that matters incredibly to us. The moments of passionate self-expression — that is the music.

A patient who sells computer components brought me roses from his garden. The look on his face as he spoke about the joyous work he did to create these beautiful flowers told the story. There was both serenity and passion in that moment for him.

"As we have seen, it is [our core being] linked inseparably to the essential creativity of life. That creativity springs from the self-organizing capacity of all living systems"[2] These are the words of an optimistic physicist, Danah Yohar. She assures us that our souls have the capacity to bring order and coherence out of our chaos. Creative self-expression is our best path to re-enchantment. It is passionate and open.

It is not a straight road that brings us to our creative soul. We shift back and forth from equilibrium to non-equilibrium because the process for all living organisms does not remain stationary. A static system is a dying one, and so we must accept the fact that we cannot have equilibrium continually. Shifts can make us more vulnerable, seeming to threaten our being and our identity, much as an earthquake threatens the integrity of plates in our cupboard. It seems we are neither here nor there for a time. It is most frightening!

When I spoke about shifting my career, I encountered a long period of non-equilibrium. Nothing sheltered me from the anxiety and vulnerability of risking. Even as I wrote (the most challenging part of my self-expression), fragmented parts of myself lay in the dust. I knew creative tension then just as Raphael knew this when he changed his medical career and Savannah knew the anxiety when she embarked on her career in music. We stepped into material that was closer and closer to our heart center, accepting the anxious, creative tension that our journeys necessitated. Remember Bron's first trip to a painting class, when she told us how difficult the forty minute ride to school was?

As our life changes and becomes chaotic, a new order appears. That new order provides a glimpse into the very essence of transformation. I briefly gave up a part of my life — therapist/guide, wife, mother, manager — and went to a verdant seashore where I wrote, walked along stretches of white beach, wet cliffs hanging over me, my feet gathering sand as I ran to retrieve a gray sand-dollar before the gulls got it. Writing, gardening, and beachcombing were my transcendence at that time. My spirit came alive within these rich experiences, but I did not always understand the significance of my passion to be at the sea writing.

During times of change it is as if I am suspended between two worlds. Murray Stein, who writes beautifully about midlife crisis and transition, describes the upheaval as liminality.

> *The English "liminality" comes from the Latin limen, meaning "doorway" or "threshold." Entering a room or leaving it, one crosses a limen, and while there, in this borderline space, one is in liminality, if only for a half second.*
>
> *In liminality the "I's" standpoint is not fixed, and it occupies no clearly defined psychological location. It floats; it is not sharply delineated as "this" and "not that"; the boundaries between "I" and "not-I" blur and come much closer together than is true in the areas of fixed psychological identity. The ego is a has been and a not-yet. Time warps: the ego forgets, the fixed edges of memory blur and fade, and the past juts forward in surprising and peculiar ways; the future has no particular image or contour. The "I" is not anchored to any particular inner images, ideas, or feelings. So, unattached, the "I" floats and drifts and wanders across many former boundaries and forbidden frontiers.*
>
> *In liminality, too, there is an unusual degree of vulnerability to sudden emotional "drafts" originating either within or without, to sudden moods and to highly charged images and thoughts, to sudden gains and losses of confidence. Inner ground shifts, and because the base is not firm, a person can be easily influenced, pushed, and blown about. A sudden*

> *happening will make a more than normally deep impression, like an imprinting. More malleable in liminality than otherwise, a person may carry the effect of such imprintings through the rest of a lifetime.*[3]

M. Stein has described what we experience when we are in transition, an interim space where we leave something that has been important and known and then embark on the unknown. We are on the threshold about to move to the other side. Because our feet are not firmly planted on new ground, the interim is a floating, emotionally vulnerable space, clearly and fearfully unbalancing for a time. Our spirit is being pulled to a future place, beyond the familiar life we know so well.

At one point in my life I chose to sculpt even while believing I had little artistic skill. When I saw a friend's work in marble, I knew I had to create in this medium. My hands ran over the smooth stone, an abstract female torso. Just then, my friend described how she learned her skills at a local college. I knew in that moment I would work on stone, whatever change this required of me. I sculpted for several years and felt joyous during the process. Selling my work was another matter, devoid of creative energy for me. Much later I decided to write. I had even less confidence in my writing ability than I had when I began sculpting. I had a comfortable wide chair in my bedroom, overlooking a desert wash filled with rabbits and quail. One spring day I grasped a yellow pad and began writing. I never stopped.

In midlife several *voices* and I experienced much turmoil. The thresholds at ages forty through sixty were by far the most difficult I had negotiated in my life. "Midlife crisis turns persons inside out and tears up their crafted worlds."[4] Unremembered dreams, visions, unconscious awareness, and our intuitive voices can guide us toward our transcendence even while we are experiencing the worst midlife chaos. Sometimes we go forward kicking and screaming, sometimes meditative and in solitude; sometimes we utilize outside resources such as therapy, somehow, some way, we clear our way to a richer reality.

When we are in chaos, old holes and voids push us against the wall, expanding our fears and anxiety. Raphael spoke to me about some thresholds he crossed while restoring his lost spirit. This is his story as I remember it:

> *His early years were a nightmare, sometimes a desperate struggle, since the negatives of childhood greatly impacted his lack of confidence. Because his mother and father constantly invaded his boundaries and were critical of his many life choices, he felt molded, un-empowered, and unaccepted. These feelings so permeated his spirit that he believed that he got into college and medical school only because his father pulled strings and got others to help Raphael achieve his goals. There had been few experiences in Raphael's early years to prove to him that he was capable or that he could be self-sufficient. These years were his chaos. Though he won a scientific award when graduating elementary school, and several scientific awards in high school and college, those positive experiences could not override his feelings of inadequacy. In high school, one mentor, in particular, believed in Raphael's abilities, believed in him as a totally independent person. This teacher supported his ambition to become a scientific researcher.*
>
> *When Raphael passed his medical specialty boards three thousand miles away from his father, he at last knew for certain that his knowledge was his own. Moving away from family and establishing his reputation solidified his sense of possessing a strong core self. He experimented with new ideas,*

but not until becoming an expert in invitro fertilization did he realize his own restorative process. Finally he had accomplished something his father could not claim he had done first, or better. That was one major transition in many long roads to re-enchant his lost spirit, and he was now well into midlife. Raphael's world during his middle years was satisfying unlike many other voices. Raphael found peace in becoming what he wanted and needed to be. He felt he grew up and gained self-respect in his midlife. He heard his music.

Beyond the customary borders of my everyday self may be new creative ambitions, different forms of self-expression. These will consciously or unconsciously call out to me to be expressed and will be satisfied as long as I am unwilling to be the *walking dead.* I accept the risks and the vulnerability, and I grieve for my previously malnourished spirit. Reluctantly, I permit myself to leave old patterns, places, careers, and people. Prima materia, the first, the passionate, richer material, becomes the most important path for me to follow. My heart encourages me to pursue my dream as I am pulled to a future place.

Where did the heart center lead the *voices*? What was the dream they pursued? Emily built a small, pure, beautiful chapel on a desert ranch far from the nearest town of eight hundred people. It is built out of straw adobe, strong and enduring. Painted walls, church altars, candles, pictures, beautiful objects adorn the simple poetic structure.

Cassi is fully engaged in a new career. She will travel extensively, bringing her the kind of adventure she has dreamed about.

Heather, living alone now, structures her daily life so that she can enjoy listening to music as well as choosing other things she wants and loves to do. She gardens, volunteers her time to political organizations, and keeps an active correspondence with her large family.

Savannah, while writing and teaching a life design program to advance people's creativity, currently composes and plays her own music in small club venues.

Bron painted several large canvases in a New York studio recently and they represent her emotional freedom.

Shana and I walk a long stretch of sand beach, watch white-capped waves in settled blue-green rows as we ponder life issues and our personal renewals. We gaze now and then at the continuity of an infinite sea, sharing thoughts, which both of us will later write. We share the idea that our lives will mirror the changes of our beloved sea, both serene and tempestuous. Shana has become CEO and owner of a small but challenging company that requires her fine entrepreneurial skills.

Amy has just installed her seven large paintings in their permanent home, a large medical center dedicated to helping women heal serious illness. At this same time she is also exhibiting a new series of paintings in galleries on both the East and West coasts.

Crossing over our thresholds, or "limens," may require major sacrifices or losses. Karen, a close friend, was busy enjoying the child she had always wanted. At last, she felt, she was hearing her music. After this wonderful event in her life, the birth of her child, she expressed dismay when her mood shifted to enormous sadness. She said, "I shouldn't be having these feelings, I want them to stop." She is grieving lost themes, lost parts of herself, as she crosses this new threshold of parenthood. These changes in her life have created conflicts with old ambitions and ideals, though the cherished gift of her child remains uppermost in her heart. At the birth of her child Karen partially gave up a demanding sales career. She feels the absence of her career like a wrenching from her deepest soul. No question, she did sacrifice a part of herself when she gave up an ego-satisfying career. "The ego needs to let go of this attachment ... preliminary to a deeper discovery of the Self ... the person needs to "find the corpse' and then to bury it."[5]

Karen asked me about her feelings of loss. Some of the ambition she felt in her work as an advertising executive was slipping away, while her new life as a mother had not yet become solid. As a sales advertising executive, Karen lived every day in crisis and anxiety even though she was the top producer in her company. There is no doubt that stepping onto the threshold between career and motherhood opens the door to a deep vulnerability. What she finally knows is that she cannot step back into the old world of ego expectations, and similar goals. Karen has a future destiny. Again and again rich dreams and fantasy illuminate this new path, but she needs time to restore her authentic self and bring her focus to her new life. Like the exotic cactus, small pieces wither and fall away while new limbs grow to balance the remaining ones. Karen will find the new ground between work and motherhood, and when she does the sense of foreboding and loss will lessen or vanish altogether.

Karen asked me a thought-provoking question: Were some abandoned work goals "outworn parts" of her self? Or were they "unfinished possibilities?" Karen did relinquish old worn-out parts of her developing career and some of her potentials were left unfinished. Both losses are acceptable. Unfinished potentials may remain the next creative markers on the road she travels.

During my midlife, when I began to discuss shifting my career to psychotherapy, my husband and some friends expressed grave concerns about giving up my art consulting business. Their advice was an aggressive expression of the possible dire consequences of making this change. Standing on the threshold between these two careers I tottered back and forth over several months, finally letting go of all external advice. "The feeling is one of alienation, marginality, and drift"[6] for me. My inner voice refused to relinquish a dream of what I wanted to be because I knew there were unfinished parts of my self waiting to be expressed. I chose to become a therapist.

There is rarely a point in time when exterior forces will stop shoving, pushing, and nudging me in directions that assault my authentic self. In fact, these outside forces seems to support and empower my internal dialogue of self-doubt and fear. Sometimes I feel like shoving back, perhaps knocking everything down. When I step over a threshold, I don't want someone standing in my face. No one denies how demanding it is to place the second foot firmly on the other side of a limen. Our spirit has enough strength to resist most forces that invade our personal space. Here we are and here we will stay, if that is our determined choice.

I am reminded about the sense of failure we can feel when we can't shift our weight to the new space on the other side of the threshold. Sara, a friend of mine since our college years, spoke to me about her despair. She believed that time had run out for her. Her ambitions and goals to be an attorney were realized but the rewards of this profession fell short of her personal expectations to be a happy, practicing lawyer. At each juncture, she placed one foot on new ground, only to retreat two steps back. At age fifty, her notion of her failure prevented her from imagining that she had any creative choices. She was mired in joyless legal work. "Nearing the ultimate decline, we ask ourselves whether we have been true to our innermost design. This is the time of utmost hopelessness for some, of utter lethargy . . . which overtakes those who feel they have failed and cannot remedy the failure in the time and with the energies still at their disposal."[7] Then Sara had a big breakthrough. She found therapist/guides who helped her reverse the process — now two steps forward, one step back. The grand illusion of her life had been a belief she would be a happy, successful lawyer. With her therapist's help she discovered being an attorney would not satisfy her own inner needs.

For thirty years she had been entertaining a dream that was as far removed from her passionate true self as a dream could be. If becoming an attorney was not her dream, what was? What would satisfy who she truly is as she moved into her middle years? She began to get the answers she'd been seeking. She discovered the vision that had been waiting for her all the while.

Sara purchased a small bookstore. She had always loved reading, and that passion led her to the joy of sharing books with her friends and customers. She also loves music, which became easy to incorporate into her store by adding a section of tapes and CD's. Through the book store, Sara established new relationships, and married within a year.

Sara's story tells us that work, love, and play can always be transformed and it is rarely too late. In fact, age can become our ally since we have greater awareness of our mortality and, like Sara, we have a formidable drive to express our deepest self.

Destiny and mortality are not immutable even when serious illness threatens me. I am a cancer survivor. Illness is a road like all other roads, with thresholds similar to others I have chosen to travel. Profound changes can be achieved during physical illness and some of us will discover work, love, and play more in tune with our transcendent spirit. When we are seriously ill, we require experiences that satisfy only our most cherished needs.

Emily shared this story about her illness and a discovery about her choices:

EMILY: My brother, the doctor, said, "Emily, the reason that you're not sleeping is because of the band-aids™ that you have been using to suppress everything." It was documented that from the day of the general surgery, I did not sleep. Band-aids™ came loose with the anesthesia. He said, "There is something that must be bothering you, you better find out what it is." He said that I should go to a psychiatrist or a psychologist, which, of course, was the farthest thing from anything I'd ever done in my life. I didn't grow up around this with my mother or my father. I am holistic, always have been, yet I didn't want to grow any more tumors.

Then a month later, I found out that I had a frozen shoulder. The doctor said that the next stage of pain would be called mental amnesia and I wouldn't be aware of my own body. He couldn't believe that I hadn't been in there sooner.

I think your body gets weak and when it gets weak, everything falls apart. This was very traumatic. I decided that this was never going to happen to me again. The only way that I could not have this happen or at least try not to have it happen, was to change my life.

Emily speaks about "band-aids™," a temporary means to suppress what she will not consciously address. She refused to experience negative feelings, to confront the issues with the significant people in her life. Her anger dropped away like a hot marshmallow from a burning skewer. If you've ever roasted marshmallows, you know they stick to your fingers. In this way emotions stick and burn. We can't just drop them; remnants remain, remnants that cause pain and confusion. Emily has developed expressive resources now, and is no longer acting out her role as the stoic pillar of strength. While playing her part as the strong one for family and friends, she withheld her own negative responses. Emily is a communicator, but she decided not to disturb anyone close to her with communication about difficult, or so-called unhappy emotions. It took great physical pain to get past her threshold of resistance. Emily now shares her emotional thoughts and feelings appropriately, but to do this, to open to this part of her life, she had to give up the pillar of strength role.

As we attempt to restore our embattled spirits our bodies may desert us. Our restoration to authenticity becomes more difficult when spirit and body fall apart at the same time. The strength to enter transformational thresholds eludes us as we marshal all our resources to heal our failing body as well as restore our dislocated spirit. Emily used the crisis of her illness to fuel necessary spiritual and mental changes she could no longer ignore. Mind, body and spirit each do best when they work together.

Physical and emotional chaos do co-exist, no doubt about it! How often have we seen someone we love — perhaps even our self — go to the edge of illness and despair? Our strengths are fragmented, and we give up doing the rich things that make our days joyful. For most of us our souls are restored one small step at a time. Within the chaos are connections and guides whose presence give us grace, lift up our spirits so that we can see our light. In a cartoon I once saw, one person was saying to another, "Look, see the light at the end of the tunnel!" In the next frame, the reader can see past the tunnel to another and another and another tunnel.

This journey we travel together doesn't change our harsh and challenging passages. But our mystical connection with each other, our mutual participation, gives us our greatest hope to restore the light, the purpose, and the joy. Albert Camus once said "To lose one's life is a little thing, and I will have the courage when necessary. But to see the meaning of life dissipate, and our reason for living disappear, that's what is unbearable."[8]

Notes to Chapter 8

1. Dag Hammerskjold, *Markings* (New York: Random House, 1964), p. 19.
2. Danah Yohar, *The Quantum Self* (New York: William Morrow and Company, Inc., 1990), p. 221.
3. Murray Stein, *In Midlife* (Texas: Spring Publishers, Inc., 1983-1986), p. 9.
4. Ibid., p. 1.
5. Ibid., p. 27.
6. Ibid., p. 9
7. Heinz Kohut, *The Restoration of the Self* (New York: International Universities Press, 1977), p. 241.
8. Albert Camus, *A Life* (New York: Alfred A. Knopf, Inc., 1997) pg. 212.

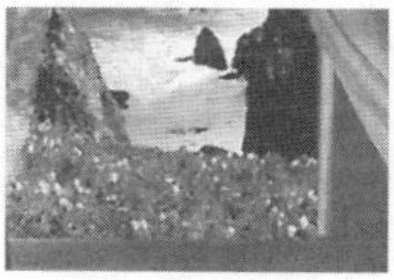

CHAPTER 11

Re-Enchantment

You have probably seen some of those Persian rugs from Tabriz that represent the Tree of Life, with every kind of creature, birds, animals, and even human beings resting in its branches. Well, when I paint, I feel as if the sap were rising from the very roots of this Tree of Life to one of its topmost branches, where I happen or try to be, and then surging through me to transform itself into forms and colors on my canvas. It is as if I were but a kind of medium, capturing or transmitting the vibrations of all that is, or that is not, in the world.

EDWARD RODITE[1]

AS CHILDREN WE STRUGGLE TO FIND OURSELVES, struggle to feel safe. I remember thinking, around age eight, how different I was from my girlfriend who lived across the street. The library was several blocks away from us, and I walked there every week, returning to my home with tales of rescued heroines. My friend had no interest in books. She was not a curious person, and she was most often lighthearted, easy, hardly aware of her continual family crises. Even then, I brooded about who I was and what would become of me. I fantasized about being a heroine in a world that was predictable. My parents had little understanding of either my real or fantasy life and my mother did not know how to provide a sense of safety, so when I turned to her, or my father, for confirmation that all was well, nothing echoed back to me. The reassurance of safety I greatly craved had been missing since my infancy. Anxiety became a lifetime companion. We moved from the city to a small town when I was nine years old. It was here that I began to experience a sense of stability for the first time in my young life. My new friends and their families became guides and loving mentors — but the original well of loneliness persisted on some core level of my soul. I know the first eight years of my life created a void I would forever try to fill. That void of emotional abandonment is a mystery I have begun to solve only in the past six years. With some deeper understanding I am more protected from this hole in my psyche than at any other time in my life.

"The environment which used to be experienced as threateningly close, is now experienced more and more as threateningly distant; where children were formerly overstimulated by the emotional life of their parents, they are now often *under stimulated*."[2] My childhood occurred during a time in history when parents were overly attentive, but for me family life contained emotional voids, a distant father who worked long hours away from home, and a mother, barely twenty years old, who was pre-occupied with her own emotional survival. I was clearly an under-stimulated and under-supported child.

Children growing up today often experience vast emotional voids created by one or both parents' working, highly stressed mothers, and missing or emotionally distanced fathers whose emotional, moral, and physical participation in the child's life is minimal. Help is not provided by siblings, extended family members, or the community. Many young children today must compete with others for any love and caring that are available, to whatever degree these may be accessible to them. Emotional and moral mayhem exaggerate their own pre-existing dark shadows, deepening holes from which their ascent becomes increasingly difficult.

My parents did provide strong moral guidance. I was certainly given ethics and a conscience (though an over-developed one) by my mother, and later by my father, who modeled strict right and wrong concepts. In this important area of my life, my parents truly did not abandon me. They insisted on my being an ethical person. I remember on one of my first days in public school, I took a friend's hair barrette. My parents levied a quick judgment and punishment.

I came across the following story, which greatly moved me and triggered some powerful feelings within me. Today in the world, there is a horrific lack of conscience, unknown during the years of my growing up. Moral chaos exists for all the participants, perpetrators and non-violent witnesses as well. I believe the events in this story moved unrelentingly to a tragedy because of a fierce moral and emotional abandonment by the family and community of those who acted. Here is the story of Deletha Word's short life.

> DETROIT: *"As dozens of onlookers cheered, three men pulled a woman from her car, stripped her to her underwear, then chased her until she either jumped or was forced off a bridge to her death.*
>
> *None of the forty or so passersby tried to help Deletha Word during the confrontation. The incident began with two minor traffic accidents early Saturday on the Belle Isle bridge, said police Sgt. John Morel.*
>
> *A man who arrived late tried to rescue her from the Detroit River but couldn't reach her. The thirty-three year-old woman's body, missing a leg, was found several miles downstream later that morning.*

"My baby was down there all by herself. I know she was scared to death," the woman's mother, Dortha Word, said as she cried Monday. "How could they be so cruel?"

The trouble started about 3 A.M.*, Morel said, when Word was involved in two minor traffic accidents on Belle Island. One car with three men inside chased her onto the bridge connecting the island to the city and rammed her car, forcing her to stop.*

One of the men smashed her car with a crowbar and pulled her from the car, ripping off some of her clothes, Cmdr. Gerald Stewart said. The man pushed her against the car and beat her.

One of the men weighed nearly 300 pounds, according to a police source quoted in The Detroit News. Word, who was 4 feet, ll inches, weighed 115 pounds, her mother said.

When Word tried to run away, police said, the man with the crowbar chased her. What happened after that is unclear.

Police would not say whether Word jumped or was forced off the bridge, but her mother said she was sure her daughter was forced into the Detroit River.

"They . . . made her leap over that bridge and beat her hands. She was holding onto the bridge, and beat her hands away from that banister," she said, citing an account she said police gave her.

Deletha Word's cousin, Carol Neely, said Word never would have jumped because she did not know how to swim.

Lawrence Walker, twenty-one, was in the bumper-to-bumper traffic that had formed on the bridge when he noticed a crowd running to the edge. He got out of his car and followed, then jumped into the river after her.

"I wasn't trying to be Superman or anything," he said. "I just saw something and jumped in without thinking about it."

But Word moved away from him and a friend in the water, and he quickly lost sight of her. He worried afterward that perhaps she thought he was one of the people after her.

"I think my trying to help her maybe made her swim a little further out than she could," he said.

Walker said about fifty people were gathered when he ran up, many of them laughing about the men beating Word. He said one person had a cellular phone but would not call police. "It seemed like people didn't care," he said.

By Sunday afternoon, police had arrested three men, two age twenty and one age nineteen. It was not clear what charges they faced.

Relatives described Word as the backbone of their close-knit family. She had a thirteen year-old daughter and worked at a grocery store while earning a bachelor's degree in marketing. When her brother, James, was shot to death in May, she was the family's support.

"If she had been on that bridge, and somebody was beating somebody, she wouldn't have stood and watched," Dortha Word said. "She would have helped them. She might have got hurt trying, but she would have helped."[3]

Who are these perpetrators? Who are the witnesses watching a young woman beaten and driven to her death? Would you recognize them if you met them in other circumstances? What holes in their spirits led to this tragedy?

Looking back, the *voices* and I acknowledge relationships with wounding and wounded families. No matter how much we may have separated ourselves, moved on, we can easily recall the terrible pain of faulty critical reflections, outright rejection, unempathetic parents telling us both verbally and nonverbally, "you are not enough," one powerful legacy of our life.

So what is the difference that allows so many of us to be decent, vital, creative, moral adults? I believe the child becomes an adult without a conscience — empty, and disturbed — because of a severely damaging childhood, but more importantly because there is little or nothing beyond the family to change the course of events. Parental failure, moral and emotional abandonment, are often passed on from one generation to the next. Now the community itself appears to exacerbate the development of a fragmented, immoral, and empty self.

I did not have models in my life to nurture my self-esteem. Moreover, in my early adulthood I made poor choices, probably based on my self-image, that diminished my sense of self-worth. I lacked self-confidence. Even though I was taught a strict ethical code, my parents, in their innocence, defaced some part of me. All the *voices,* as we've learned, also experienced some similar negative influences. Yet, because of a strength provided by a deeper source, perhaps a tangled wing of our genetic nature, or more positive later world experiences, we survived the mayhem. I may never be able to determine what part of this strength was genetic and what part was environmental, but I took something essential, something human, something creative from these and became a decent person. I found links to restore my dislocated, lost spirit. They are my fiercely guarded internal capacity for accomplishment, and external sources of strength and love. I sought them out and insisted on their presence in my life. And the *voices,* as well, demanded creative solutions to the mysteries of their lives. They heard their own music.

Savannah was deprived of emotionally supportive parents. She described how her father divorced her mother, and abandoned her morally and emotionally, at the beginning of her life. Her mother, Ellen, left alone, was sorely inadequate to raise three children. She found escapes in several addictive substances. Ellen withdrew from all semblance of a vital life, years before her actual suicide.

Savannah developed a strong moral code to be "the good girl," thinking it would help her mother. For a long period of her life (until she left for New York), she blocked her creativity by complying with what she thought to be the shoulds, the I-must-do-list of a good girl. During those early years she took care of everybody but herself. Much later, after pursuing a career in music and enduring many difficult transitions, she built powerful love, work, play, and creative structure. Earlier in this chapter, she told her story of the experiences of a vulnerable, fragile and, at times, empty self, and now she provides a memoir of thoughts and experiences that helped her reclaim her lost spirit.

> **SAVANNAH: I studied Shamanism twenty years ago. I was a yogi for twenty-five years. The ability to meditate was a very strong structure for me. I think in retrospect it was another way to escape, but it was also a strong thread that gave me strength.**
>
> **I had to break the rules enough to touch into my authenticity. The way that I context that is that in order to touch into the part of me that I had disowned, the missing creativity, I had to dance with the devil, which means I had to embrace my fear, and my fear was in ever doing anything wrong. That was my greatest fear.**
>
> **I used my mind to justify being able to go for my heart. The first thing that came up was all of this intellectual and spiritual information. I was able later to get grounded enough to open up my system and begin the work of the heart. I actually began that in the summer of 1982 when I did my first past life therapy session. Those were the first**

feelings that I had. Since that time, I have opened up more and more of those flood gates and now I am in touch with my emotional nature. I see that as a gift, as a natural flow of things, the juice of life, the catalyst for my creativity.

When I was in the era of gaining all that intellectual insight into my spiritual nature, gleaning that information which was opening the doors, I thought that was the transcendence. In a way, it's part of the process of transcending, but it's only the beginning. It's when I could really get it in my emotional being that it truly started shifting who I am and how I perceive the world and how the world perceives me.

Shifting itself is transcendent. When we can be in that constant shifting with emotion and comfort, we are transcendent.

"Magic is the ability to change consciousness at will." We create the shift. Understanding that we are making it up by what we call it. The positioning itself is the creative dynamic, it's that we know we're making it up. How we position it is how it ends up.

"Shift Happens" is Savannah's bumper sticker

Years of intellectual, emotional, and spiritual data gathering led to an opening of Savannah's emotional life, and a revitalization of her heart center. Only then did her rich, creative material flow. The music she wrote and recorded came from the depths of her soul, from crisis and transitions, from grief, from loss, from all the spirit's emotional work. Savannah viewed herself as anxious, needing comfort about changing her life. She was able to see these times of anxious transition as creative tension. Design, art, performing music, and teaching life-design seminars now brings a great sense of abundance to her life. If she had not accepted the anxiety and tension, her work would not have been productive and joyful.

I believe what Savannah shares about creative tension and positioning is very important. Transcendent beings welcome their transitions. She views her transitional times *as a creative challenge accompanied by anxiety.* This new label or positioning is everything, because when we label something we are making it this thing, not that, and too easily it becomes a self-fulfilling prophecy, as Savannah says, "how it ends up."

Savannah is hardly alone in walking her path of fear. I have clear pictures of my own fears. In my mind, I can scan all the old events that frightened me. I know many of these demons extremely well, and now, after considerable work, I am able to penetrate the mysteries surrounding them. I engage my rational mind by asking some questions. What control do I possess, since my worst fear is being unable to control events. One of my old myths was that I could control almost anything. If there are steps where I can take control, I organize the actions that will produce a better comfort level. My thoughts are focused at this point on each step, and my feeling of fear is diminishing. If what I am afraid of is not within my control, I make a great effort to release that fear and accept my destiny. I am learning to trust the outcome, and to believe that all I need will be provided.

Strong mentors conveyed to me a powerful understanding that I can live without being too invested in or troubled by the outcome of events that are beyond my control. I can trust that whatever happens is meant to be and controlling or forcing the outcome is not the answer. If I am always invested in one particular solution, I lose the ease and joy of my journey. There is no logical basis for trust. I know that. It is a leap of faith and I ask my spirit to take that leap because it provides the best hope I have to live more serenely, to experience the texture of events unclouded by fear.

Flying is a good example of my giving up control. Since I do not know how to fly the plane or make decisions, my anxiety is greatly increased during flights. It is the one demon causing me to work the hardest at acceptance and release of fear. During a turbulent flight I am not always successful at diminishing my fears, but I am much better with trust. I have stopped checking the weather. Often I enjoy the clouds and lights below. That is a recent gift.

What strikes me profoundly about anxiety and fear is our ability to change it, to release ourselves from a legacy of a crumbling self, held captive by the weight of these damaging, emotional affects. Distinct from the use of drugs that dull the feelings, the development of trust, regardless of the outcome, can inspire an enormous shift away from fear.

When I spoke about fear and the voids, some themes of my book, someone asked me why I chose the particular ten voices that I did. There are at least two answers to this question. There was a wonderful play and movie titled *Six Degrees of Separation.* The theme is that we are separated from each other by only six people; therefore, we are more connected to everyone in the universe than we ordinarily recognize. Perhaps the *voices* I know so well are one means for the readers to recognize the connection of themselves to another. As Camus wrote, we may all be on "a parched road to hope." It comforts the soul to know we are not alone. Guides arrive in many forms and some may be here in these *voices.* That is the second reason for my choice.

Amy's heart closed down and her world grew dark. Her autoimmune illness kept her bedridden much of the day, and then a shift occurred. She sat up one morning and knew her physical treatments had imperceptibly brought about change in her strength. With almost no energy, she began to attend a group that met daily to share spiritual teachings. The healing began with that small group of people, and progressed during the next two years. She renewed her life and it took a different form because she no longer drives herself to the point of exhaustion. Her daily life is calmer, quieter, focused on an inner vision of what she wants to accomplish. She carefully chooses those things that fulfill her passionate needs. If it's not primary, it's discarded. Her choices are not always harmonious. There are days when she cannot fulfill even her simplest goals and some of her illusions about strength still trouble her. The remarkable fact is that Amy is recovering. She is painting for a show, and she participates more in her life than she could have imagined one year ago.

To be part of a our richer, larger spirit sometimes requires work that digs into unconscious awareness. Our spirit needs to know and accept the dark shadow, the Swiss cheese holes of our psyches, the voids we attempt to fill with compensatory choices. Early on, mysteries embedded in our souls, mysteries that developed with the twists of life events, need to be solved.

WHO, WHEN, WHERE, HOW . . . FULLER AWARENESS OF THESE QUESTIONS BRINGS US TO A WINDOW OF UNDERSTANDING. WHO WAS PRESENT? WHEN DID THE MYSTERY BEGIN? TO THE BEST OF MY MEMORY, WHERE WAS I? HOW DID I PERCEIVE THE MYSTERY THEN? HOW DO I PERCEIVE IT NOW?

Emily solved her partially unconscious mystery of when and how her father emotionally abandoned her. She forgave her father his tennis torture after learning many facts about his obsessive illness and she uncovered more personal memories about their good times together. Her creativity, work, love, and play enable her to step beyond the past dark shadows of her childhood. Creativity is the persistent essence of her vastly richer self.

In midlife Raphael understood and forgave his mother, now age ninety-one, both her benign neglect and her active destruction of normal boundaries. He was able to love his father in spite of the competitive themes and feelings of inadequacy that he imposed on his son. Raphael searched out family information by meeting several times with an aunt who knew all his family's secrets. He gained wisdom about his parent's relationship and the history of previous generations, especially as it was affected by his maternal grandparents. He was able to put together a tapestry of knowledge that led to grace and forgiveness.

In her youth, Bron's mother had been responsible for raising her own brothers and sisters, and she clearly didn't want to parent her own two children. That information helped answer some of the questions Bron had about who, when, why, and how Bron herself was emotionally abandoned. Years of self-exploration and therapy brought to light some of Bron's deepest questions about her own mysterious voids. She moved from the shadows of unrequited mother-love to an experience of mutual nurturing with her own husband, son, and daughter.

Shana had unusual powers of observation, even as a child, to intuitively understand pieces of her mystery. She could accept her father's limitations to perceive her as an adult since she discovered he needed to preserve the happier time in his own life when she was a child. Shana suffered because her visions and dreams that foretold the future frightened some people. Her family and friends were put off by her vision of different levels of spiritual worlds. She found a solution to the primary mystery of why and how people rejected her for her differences. In her own life she embraced ideals and principles of unconditional love, non-judgment, and acceptance of every being as a divine essence. As she did so, she broke through her isolation. Also, the world changed and people became curious and more open-minded about multi-dimensional reality. The fact is, Shana opened doors to that mystery for me and many others to see. I will never understand all that Shana envisions, but I *see* more and more for myself as a result of her influence in my life.

Kay's box, given to her by her father during her childhood, served her well, since it provided a serious, continuous response to all her mysteries. The box proscribed ethics and principles of living and these were a foundation for her innately caring and determined nature. If the box were not provided, her response to being born with a spinal defect could have negatively impacted her capacity for living her life fully. Kay participates in her life, with few reservations.

Cassi knows some of the mystery of her parents' and grandparents' life-design, especially her grandmother's worldview of responsibility and freedom. She knows what is important to accomplish for herself and believes in her freedom and her power to do it. She has moved to the East Coast to further her career. That move separated her physically from her family, but she remains emotionally connected to them, especially to her mother. This family support gives Cassi strength to respond in highly effective ways to difficult challenges. Both work and love are now in transition and some of the mystery concerning her personal relationships persist even today.

Tina began to change her life after being raped. She sought therapy to get past the horrific event and she also called upon Native American Spirit ancestors who helped her walk the way, surefooted up a mountain path. Tina's metaphor was small steps from one camp to another, like those who climb the upper reaches of Mt. Everest. Frequent storms prevailed in her climb, preventing her from advancing for long periods of time. But she always envisioned the next camp. She learned to speak and live with her authentic voice. And then, a serious illness devastated both her self-respect and her strength. Her music stopped. She now courageously fights for survival, remembering her music by recreating all the emotional and mental support she has experienced in the past. Every day Tina calls up the spirit of re-enchantment and she asks her Native American ancestors to join her in a quest to better manage the lengthening shadows of illness and despair. Rituals old and new guide her gently back to loving herself.

Heather struggles for independence and freedom. The largest mystery in her life was why freedom didn't exist for her. Within the tight confines of a shared home with her sister, every day brought a new campaign to preserve her own space. She is, at age sixty-eight, weary beyond her years, yet she functions by aiding her favorite charities, listening to music she loves, and planting flowers, the latter being symbols of her passion and creativity. The burdens of doctors' appointments, medicine, frequent trips to the market for food, and daily tasks of maintenance have become her life. But her life, amidst some lost dreams, is also connection, small acts of kindness, generosity, and love. Just recently her sister has moved to her own apartment, and Heather blossoms with her newfound freedom. Understanding her emotional attachment to her sister (one mystery) enabled Heather to let go of a damaging relationship for both sisters.

Solving our mysteries, understanding the voids, is essential. Even when we do this, others rush to judgment. People will often say, I can't believe so-and-so was ever in therapy; she is such a mess, or her life is so miserable! Or they will say, how can he make such bad decisions, he's had so much therapy? The judgments implied in all the questions are certainly inappropriate, but something much more fundamental exists. When we view another's life we have no notion of what has impacted that person, perhaps from the moment of their conception. Even when we are involved intimately, we can not always understand the miracle of their achievements as they relate to all their mysteries. At best we see the tip of the iceberg. Re-enchantment of their lost spirit would be a miracle under any circumstances and if we have a clear view of all that has gone before, the miracle is even more remarkable.

Melvin Konner, author and speaker, tells a story about being taken to a museum of natural history by one of his college professors:

> *There I met a man who had devoted most of his life to the study of the skeletal remains of archaeopteryx — the earliest tetrapod with feathered wings — embedded in a Mesozoic rock. I was introduced to him, awed by him, impressed with his intelligence and wisdom. It was obvious that he wanted to impart to me some piece of genuine, useful knowledge gained from the countless hours of squinting over that crushed tangle of bone and rock.*
>
> *What he finally said was that he thought archaeopteryx was very much like people. This of course puzzled me, as it was calculated to do, and when I pressed him to explain, he said, "Well, you know, it's such a transitional creature. It's a piss-poor reptile, and it's not very much of a bird."*[4]

Ask yourself, just as the *voices* and I did — Raphael, Emily, Bron, Shana, Amy, Cassi, Kay, Tina, Heather, and Savannah: If I speak about restoring my lost soul, what stories will I tell? Is it a story about voids within myself? Is it about a life-design I could not develop or maintain, work and love that died? Is it a story about what might have been? Opportunities lost? Is it a story about living within the dark shadows of my mind? Is it a story of spiritual and physical isolation? Or is it a story of discovery, finding work, relationships, and play that is often compelling and joyful? Is it a story about living in my heart center, living with passion, living creatively? Is it a story about my mercy and forgiveness, a reconciliation with me and those I love? Is it my story of attachment and connection? Finally, is it a story about my lost, dislocated spirit hearing, once again, my glorious music?

> **AMY: My mother was sick for many years and was very frightened. At the end, she was beginning to go crazy with her fear of being dead because she had done these things to us. At the end, I said I forgive you. She said I know you do but your sister doesn't. I called up my sister and asked her to forgive our mother and she did. My mother's face got radiant and I prayed a lot about how to help her die.**
>
> **I said I had been doing angels in the studio and they were to help her go to heaven. There's a legend in Jewish myth that every time you create a good deed in this world, you create an angel in the next world. I said "Mom, look at all the good deeds you've done in your life. So, between my angels in my studio and your angels . . . when you are ready to die, just sit up in bed and put your hand out and say, 'I'm ready death angel,' and all the angels that we both created will help you to heaven."**
>
> **I don't know how I got that story. It just came to me and she said that it was a wonderful story but that she was**

> **in no rush. I flew home and did the angel of deliverance and I knew she would die because it had a skull on the side of its head and it looked like a death mask.**
>
> **She died the next day and, when I flew home, I said to the nurse, how did she die? And the nurse said she was very peaceful after my visit. She sat up in bed at 5:15 A.M. and she said to the nurse, "I'm ready, do you want to go with me?" The nurse said, "No, you won't be sick anymore with the angels." And my mother said, "Well, I'm ready death angel." She put out her hand just like my painting and she died.**

If I believe that my life and the life of others around me was not about struggling with holes and voids from birth on, it would be a cruel illusion. Our genetic natures, families, and experiences provide a destiny of continual work in order for us to maintain dignity and self-worth. We restore our lost, dislocated spirit many times during our lives, and we accomplish this with creative, passionate, authentic choices. When we are successful, work, love, and play bring joy and abundance to us. The miracle is that we can change our destiny by facing the voids. Albert Camus, an extraordinary man and writer, says "There is vertigo in losing oneself and denying everything, in breaking forever what once defined us, and which now offers only solitude and the void, all in order to find the only platform from which destinies may always begin again."[5]

Transcendence is our soul becoming a miracle of self-expression, living a richer, more passionate existence, always guided by our truest heart.

I may create a life that seems maddening, just beyond my outstretched hand, and from this existence, disappointments that could kill my soul. What I want is a *small shift* to a personal vision of what I can be, a small step to being alive and joyful. What makes a difference for the *voices* and me, is this remarkably simple and small shift in our daily destiny.

Do you believe the myth that you are alone as you fight fiercely to restore your lost spirit? All that you are is in some form struggling within other souls, six degrees of separation, you and I and the *voices* journeying together. We transform something in our lives every day, and each day we go forward with a small, sometimes imperceptible change. As I sit writing, the oak leaves fall out of season, some trees shedding their dying, gray, unwelcome leaves, as other shoots are already showing themselves soft, velvet, green emeralds on gray branches.

Small steps follow one upon another — work, play, creativity, joy, purpose, love, attachment, passion. A lightening bolt of recognition rarely hits me. I have a brief awareness, a dim light of insight, an intuitive foretelling, a hand holding my hand warmly as I grope toward hope. "*The Tree of Life where I happen or try to be.... It is as if I were but a kind of medium capturing or transmitting the vibrations of all that is, or that is not in the world.*"[6]

Off in the distance I can hear a flute playing. I know these sounds so well. Words accompany the music and I speak them softly to you.

"There is a meeting place, a crossing over where heaven and earth weave wholeness, and balance is restored.... This is the migration home, and the connection rests on a blade of grass...."[7]

Notes to Chapter 11

1. Edward Rodite, *Dialogues on Art* (As referenced in a private journal), p. 207.

2. Heinz Kohut, *The Restoration of the Self* (New York University Press, 1977), p. 271.
3. *The Oregonian,* August 22, 1995, pp. A1, A7.
4. Melvin Konner, *The Tangled Wing: Biological Constraints on the Human Spirit* (New York: Harper and Row, 1982), pp. 434 — 435.
5. Albert Camus, *A Life* (New York: Alfred A. Knopf, Inc., 1997), p. 252.
6. Edward Rodite, *Dialogues on Art* (As referenced in a private journal), p. 207.
7. *Migrations,* Ia Tulip, Sedona Arizona (a self-produced musical tape).

How to Contact the Author

As a guide through your journey to re-enchantment, the author is available for personal or couple consultation. She is also available for seminars.

Visit the author at her Website
selfdiscoveryofspirit.com

Order copies of the book, or write to Dr. Zell-Tamis at
Beverleesee4ever@aol.com

Phone: 602-956-4073

Fax: 602-952-6779

Quantity discounts are available.